MW00949084

Renal Diet Cookbook for Beginners:

Easy-to-Follow Guide by a Reputed Doctor with Tasty Low Sodium, Potassium, Phosphorus Dishes and Daily Meal Plans to Maintain Kidney Health

Dr. Tamara S. Kears

Table of Content

© Copyright 2024 by Dr. Tamara S. Kears - All rights reserved.

The following Book is reproduced below with the goal of providing information that is as accurate and reliable as possible. Regardless, purchasing this Book can be seen as consent to the fact that both the publisher and the author of this book are in no way experts on the topics discussed within and that any recommendations or suggestions that are made herein are for entertainment purposes only. Professionals should be consulted as needed prior to undertaking any of the action endorsed herein.

This declaration is deemed fair and valid by both the American Bar Association and the Committee of Publishers Association and is legally binding throughout the United States.

Furthermore, the transmission, duplication, or reproduction of any of the following work including specific information will be considered an illegal act irrespective of if it is done electronically or in print. This extends to creating a secondary or tertiary copy of the work or a recorded copy and is only allowed with the express written consent from the Publisher. All additional right reserved.

The information in the following pages is broadly considered a truthful and accurate account of facts and as such, any inattention, use, or misuse of the information in question by the reader will render any resulting actions solely under their purview. There are no scenarios in which the publisher or the original author of this work can be in any fashion deemed liable for any hardship or damages that may befall them after undertaking information described herein.

Additionally, the information in the following pages is intended only for informational purposes and should thus be thought of as universal. As befitting its nature, it is presented without assurance regarding its prolonged validity or interim quality. Trademarks that are mentioned are done without written consent and can in no way be considered an endorsement from the trademark holder.

Introduction

Welcome, dear reader, to the cradle of transformation. As a medical professional specializing in nephrology, I have witnessed the power of informed choices and positive dietary transformations on countless lives. My experiences shaping patients' journeys towards improved kidney health have been the seed that sprouted into this comprehensive guide on the renal diet.

This book is a tapestry of science, stories, and sumptuous recipes, all woven together to simplify and demystify the intricate workings of the renal diet. While our main focus may be the kidneys, the principles and ideas we'll explore are deeply rooted in overall holistic health and wellness. Navigating kidney disease is a journey filled with changes and challenges. The spectrum can be overwhelming as you grapple to grasp concepts, foods, and lifestyle adaptations drawn into the orbit of kidney health. But knowledge is your compass.

The recipe chapters are a concoction of health and flavor, carefully crafted to suit your palate while nourishing your kidneys. With each recipe, you reclaim and celebrate the joy of delicious, nutritious meals without compromising your wellbeing. The art of seasoning, mastering healthier cooking techniques, and understanding permissible and prohibited foods will become second nature to you.

Grounded in science, tempered with personal experiences, this book is the distillation of my efforts to bring the complexities of kidney health into more accessible terms. As we journey together through these pages, my hope is that you feel empowered to navigate this path courageously, full of faith in yourself and the choices you're making for your health.

BONUS PDF: To enhance your experience, we provide access to a digital version of these recipes -complete with colorful photos. Effortlessly browse these delightful recipes on your smartphone or tablet at your leisure. Scan this QR code to download them.

Chapter 1: Step Into the World of the Renal Diet

1.1. The Importance of Kidney Health

Discovering the Significance of Healthy Kidneys

Your kidneys are vital organs that play a crucial role in maintaining your body's overall health. Understanding the importance of kidney health is essential in order to ensure that you can prevent, manage, and even reverse kidney disease effectively. The primary function of the kidneys is to filter waste and excess fluids from your blood. They also help maintain the body's balance of electrolytes, regulate blood pressure, and produce hormones that control red blood cell production and bone health.

In order to maintain optimal kidney health, it is important to adopt a healthy lifestyle, exercise regularly, and follow the recommended dietary guidelines, especially for people with kidney disease or at risk of developing it. This chapter will provide an in-depth understanding of kidney health and reveal the significant role it plays in your overall well-being.

The Effects of Kidney Disease on Your Body

Kidney disease can have a profound impact on your body and overall health. When the kidneys lose their ability to function properly, waste and toxins can build up in your bloodstream. This in turn can cause symptoms like fatigue, nausea, headaches, and difficulty concentrating. As kidney disease progresses, more severe complications may arise, such as anemia, bone disease, heart disease, and even kidney failure, which might necessitate dialysis or a kidney transplant. It is crucial to address kidney disease at the earliest stage and adopt proper diet and lifestyle changes to prevent further deterioration of your kidney function.

Early Detection: The Key to Preventing Further Damage

Kidney disease often has no apparent symptoms in the early stages, and it can progress silently. This is why early detection is crucial to slow down the progression and prevent further kidney damage. Regular medical check-ups and blood tests, especially for those at risk of kidney disease (such as individuals with diabetes, hypertension, or a family history of kidney problems), play a significant role in early detection.

Once detected, a doctor will usually recommend a tailored treatment plan for each patient. This often includes dietary changes, incorporating a renal diet, managing existing health issues (like diabetes and hypertension), and making necessary lifestyle adjustments.

The Role of a Renal Diet in Kidney Health

A renal diet is specifically designed for individuals with kidney disease or people at risk of developing the condition. This diet aims to help your kidneys function more efficiently, reduce the workload on the organs, and delay the progression of the disease or even prevent it altogether in certain cases. Adopting a renal diet can make a substantial difference in managing and preventing further kidney damage.

The renal diet focuses primarily on restricting the intake of salt (sodium), potassium, and phosphorus. By limiting these key elements, you can help to ease the burden on your kidneys, as well as manage blood pressure and control the levels of other vital minerals in your body. Additionally, the renal diet promotes the consumption of healthy protein and emphasizes the importance of certain fruits, vegetables, and whole grains.

Embracing Change: The Positive Impact on Your Kidneys & Overall Health

Making the necessary changes to your eating habits and adopting a renal diet may seem difficult at first, but the benefits for your kidney health and overall well-being are immense. By following a renal diet, you not only promote better kidney function, but also lower your risk of developing other complications associated with kidney disease, such as high blood pressure and heart disease.

As you delve deeper into the world of the renal diet, you will learn how to create delicious, satisfying meals that cater to your specific dietary needs, while also ensuring that you are taking care of your kidneys. Before long, you might be surprised by the improvements you notice in your overall health, mood, and energy levels as your body responds to these positive changes.

Supporting Your Kidney Health: One Step at a Time

By understanding the importance of kidney health, acknowledging the impact of kidney disease on your body, and taking steps to adopt a renal diet, you are making a significant investment in your overall health and well-being.

This chapter marks the first step of your journey towards a healthier, happier life, and a new world of understanding and caring for your kidneys. With every page you turn, you will gain more knowledge, tips, and tools to help you manage your renal diet, prevent further kidney damage, and make informed decisions about your lifestyle.

1.2. The Benefits of a Renal Diet

The kidney is often dubbed as the silent hero of our body — working quietly, efficiently, none would expect that this pair of bean-shaped organs carries out some of the most potent tasks vital to our existence. However, when this silent hero is under threat, it calls for our immediate attention. In the quest for optimum kidney health, a powerful ally comes in the form of a renal diet.

Why is a renal diet so important? Let's delve into the myriad of benefits it offers.

Breathing Life Into Your Kidneys

A renal diet acts as a vital support system for your kidneys. It functions like a team of diligent custodians, managing and maintaining the waste and toxins that your kidneys filter out from your body. It regulates the quantity of specific nutrients your body receives, most notably sodium, potassium, and phosphorous — elements that hold the potential to strain your kidneys if allowed to escalate uncontrollably.

Key to this management is the careful regulation of protein intake. High protein consumption can burden your kidneys, but too little protein could leave your body nutritionally deficient. A well-balanced renal diet strikes the perfect harmony, introducing adequate protein into your diet without taxing your kidneys.

More Than A Kidney Ally

The benefits of a renal diet aren't confined to the kidneys; it extends a helping hand to your entire body. When we nourish our bodies with a renal diet, we're also fortifying our overall health.

For instance, contemplating high blood pressure? A renal diet is predominantly low in sodium, and maintaining a low-sodium diet helps to control hypertension, which in turn aids in minimizing kidney damage.

Concerning diabetes? Opting for an adequate amount of high-quality protein can mitigate the risk of kidney damage caused by diabetes — a condition that carries a significant risk for kidney diseases.

Similar correlations can be found between a balanced renal diet and conditions such as heart disease, osteoporosis, and malnutrition, highlighting the expansive reach of this diet's benefits.

Promoting Wellness and Positivity

Embracing a renal diet aligns you with a lifestyle that promotes a holistic sense of wellness. Healthy eating is a building block of overall well-being, supplying fuel not just for your body but also for your mind. The consciousness required to maintain a renal diet — reading nutrition labels, portion control, and incorporating diverse, colorful foods into your meals — cultivates mindfulness. This mindful eating can enhance your relationship with food, instilling a positive attitude towards nutrition while reducing overeating and binge-eating tendencies.

Moreover, a renal diet alerts us to overlooked elements in our meals and snacks. We learn to appreciate foods in their natural, unprocessed form, fostering a newfound respect for whole, nutritious foods. Learning that healthy food can be flavorful food is an enriching journey, cascading onto other aspects of your life, creating a holistic atmosphere of health-conscious behavior.

Tailoring A Taste For Life

Finally, a renal diet isn't a one-size-fits-all proposition. Just as our kidneys, despite their common functions, operate in the context of our unique bodies, a renal diet is adaptable to individual needs and conditions. This flexibility enables a renal diet to be tailored to a wide array of taste palettes and nutritional requirements.

For example, if you enjoy a robust meat dish, a renal diet can be planned to include lean protein sources. Vegetarian or vegan? You can build a renal diet incorporating plant-based proteins and other essential nutrients. The adaptability of the renal diet ensures that you don't have to abandon your preferences but learn to align them with your kidney health goals.

The beauty of a renal diet lies in its ability to be personalized. It's not an enforced regimen meant to stifle your culinary joy. Instead, it's an invitation to explore the world of flavors within the boundaries of nutritious, kidney-friendly foods.

The Renal Diet: A Lifelong Companion

Remember, kidney health, like any other aspect of our health, isn't a sprint but a marathon. It's a lifelong commitment, a journey that unfolds each passing day. The renal diet isn't a quick-fix solution or a temporary diet trend. It's here to stay, encouraging a sustained approach towards healthful eating.

The world of renal diet invites us to share in the responsibility of caring for our kidneys. The benefits of a renal diet touch every corner of our well-being — from our silent kidney heroes to our heart, our bones, and beyond. And as we take diligent strides along this path of balanced, mindful, and healthful eating — the possibility of protecting our bodies, nurturing our health, and enhancing our life quality brightly shines ahead.

Chapter 2: Know Your Food: Permitted and Prohibited

2.1. Sodium, Potassium, and Phosphorus

In our journey of kidney health, we have explored the resilient world of renal diets and their affirming benefits in our previous chapter. Now, it's time to dive deeper — to understand the roots of a renal diet, the powerhouse nutrients that shape it, starting with three critical components: sodium, potassium, and phosphorus.

The triumvirate of sodium, potassium, and phosphorus might seem nonchalant in the grandeur of all nutrients. However, they play an integral part in our diet and, even more so, in a renal diet, due to their vital roles in biological functions and their impact on kidney health.

First, let's unpack these three nutrients individually, understand their significance and limitations, and then explore their collective role in a renal diet.

Sodium: The Double-Edged Sword

Sodium, a mineral and an electrolyte, is far more than just a pillar of our common table salt. This seemingly inconspicuous nutrient is responsible for maintaining our body's fluid balance, supporting nerve and muscle function, and regulating blood pressure. Despite its importance, it stands as a double-edged sword for our health in the context of consumption.

Excess sodium can lead to fluid buildup in the body. It mimics a domino effect as this fluid buildup puts pressure on the heart and blood vessels, leading to high blood pressure. Now, here's the catch – persistent high blood pressure can cause damage to kidneys, hindering its ability to filter out wastes and toxins efficiently.

For those with compromised kidney function, the situation can be even more challenging as their kidneys find it tough to eliminate the surplus sodium, exacerbating the fluid balance and compounding health problems. The delicate line between just right and overboard is why sodium holds such critical consideration in a renal diet.

Potassium: The Essential yet Tricky Balancer

On to the next key player, Potassium - a vital mineral and also an electrolyte, responsible for many significant functions. Potassium serves to maintain fluid and electrolyte balance, regulate nerve signals, and manage muscle contractions, including the beating of our hearts.

However, as crucial as potassium is to our health, uncontrolled potassium levels can be trouble, particularly for kidneys. Healthy kidneys maintain a fine balance of potassium by eliminating excess from the blood. But when kidneys aren't functioning optimally, they may struggle to maintain this balance, leading to high potassium levels in the blood, known as hyperkalemia. This condition, if unchecked, can result in heart rhythm problems or even a heart attack. Acknowledging its importance, yet respecting its potential risks, is crucial when incorporating potassium into a renal diet.

Phosphorus: The Shadow Nutrient

Phosphorus may seem like just another nutrient on a long list, but it's uniquely important. Playing a myriad of roles, phosphorus helps build and repair bones and teeth, manage how our body stores energy, and even aid in muscle contractions.

However, phosphorus's shadow comes to light in kidney disease. Much like its other two companions, phosphorus can pose challenges when kidneys aren't functioning at their best. Excess phosphorus can't be eliminated efficiently by kidneys with impaired function, and this leads to high phosphate levels in the blood. Over time, these elevated levels can cause damage, including bone disease, arterial hardening, and even heart disease. Hence, understanding and managing phosphorus intake is crucial in a renal diet.

The Collective Impact: Balanced Intake for Renal Health

Now that we have unpacked the three elements individually, the collective role of sodium, potassium, and phosphorus in a renal diet comes to light. All three nutrients are bound by a common thread—their seemingly innocuous yet significant impact on kidney health and their need for firm and judicious regulation in a renal diet. Thus, the motto in a renal diet concerning these nutrients is lucid: Precise, prudent, and personalized moderation.

Embracing a renal diet doesn't require banishing these nutrients outright. Instead, it entails understanding their roles, acknowledging their impacts, and making sound dietary choices that offer balanced nutrition without straining the kidneys.

For instance, targeting sodium means opting for fresh foods over processed, canned, or fast foods high in salt. You can still relish the flavor by choosing spices or herbs that can add gusto to your meals without the high sodium. When it comes to potassium, a renal diet focuses on portion sizes of high-potassium foods and encourages choices with lower potassium content. Similarly, phosphorus intake could be managed by reducing consumption of certain dairy products, processed foods, and drinks laden with phosphate additives.

Remember, the goal of a renal diet isn't about sacrificing or deprivation; it's about smart moderation, about amplifying the protective and beneficial aspects of our diet while dialing down components that can pose risks. Sodium, potassium, and phosphorus — this vital nutrient trio — embodies this philosophy.

Taking its cue from the meticulous rhythm and intuition of our kidneys, a renal diet puts its faith in the power of balance and prudence. As we continue on this enriching journey of a renal diet, we shall encounter more such harmonies in our diet, learn about foods that applaud our kidney health, and discover a flavorful symphony of nutrients that sing our body's wellness.

2.2. Healthy Protein Sources

The culinary canvas of renal health is rich, diverse, and full of color. But no nutrient is perhaps as commandingly significant as protein. As we embrace this essential macronutrient's story, we move a step further in our journey of discerning renal-friendly foods. After understanding the role of Sodium, Potassium, and Phosphorus in the previous section, let's deepen our exploration, navigate the protein panorama, and understand how to select healthy protein sources for a renal diet.

Protein: The Body's Vigorous Workhorse

Protein isn't just a nutrient; it's a symphony of countless functions that lend vitality to our bodies. It plays a significant role, from building and repairing tissues, forming antibodies to fight infections, to acting as enzymes facilitating various bodily processes — the depth and breadth of protein's functions are truly astonishing.

A Balancing Act: Protein and Kidney Health

The relationship between protein and kidney health is a delicate balance, somewhat paradoxical. On the one hand, protein is crucial for good health, while on the other, excessive protein can strain the kidneys. This is because metabolizing protein produces waste, which healthy kidneys filter from the blood.

In the case of impaired kidney function, however, kidneys struggle to filter out these waste products. Therefore, an excess of protein can further burden the kidneys, as they need to work harder to eliminate the waste. However, it also should be noted that an inadequate intake of protein can lead to malnutrition, leading to further health complications. Hence, for those with kidney disease, optimal protein intake is a balancing act – not too much, not too little.

Making Wise Choices: Embracing Healthy Protein Sources

The balancing conundrum on protein intake brings us to the underlying question - how do we incorporate protein into our diet without overwhelming our kidneys? While "how much" is important, "what kind" of protein we choose plays an equally significant role.

Valuing Vitality: The Lean and Luscious Path

The dictum for choosing protein in a renal diet is to embrace lean, low-fat sources—a step that goes a long way to reduce the unnecessary strain on the kidneys and also support heart health. These sources include lean cuts of meat, skinless poultry, fish, and egg whites.

For instance, a tender, skinless chicken breast, a stalking rainbow trout fish lightly grilled, or an energizing egg-white scramble — these are not only excellent sources of protein but also incredibly versatile ingredients that can be crafted into a myriad of delicious, kidney-friendly meals.

Plant Powers: The Green Protein Route

While animal proteins are considered high-quality due to their complete amino acid profile, plant-based proteins are not to be underestimated. In fact, they can also be a valuable part of a renal diet. Certain types of plant proteins may be easier for some kidneys to process, in particular if kidney disease is advanced.

The plant kingdom offers a treasure of protein-rich foods. Think of a hearty lentil soup, a resplendent chickpea curry, or a whole-grain quinoa salad adorned with vibrant fresh vegetables — each one a testament to the power of plant proteins. Lentils, beans, and peas harbor good amounts of protein, and so do whole grains and certain seeds and nuts. However, one must be mindful of the phosphorous content of some of these options.

Tacking the Dairy Delicate

Dairy products are an excellent protein source. However, they also can be high in phosphorus and potassium, which need careful monitoring in a renal diet. But that doesn't mean they are off-limits. It is about choosing wisely. For example, certain types of cheese (like ricotta, cream cheese) and milk alternatives (like almond or rice milk) generally are lower in phosphorus and potassium, making them more kidney-friendly options.

Sensible Subtleties: The Art of Knowing Your Protein

As we discern the protein landscape, it isn't just the source of protein itself that matters but also how it is processed. For instance, preserved meats often contain high levels of sodium, which could be damaging to renal health. Similarly, certain high-protein dishes can be laden with unhealthy fats, detracting from the overall health goals of a renal diet.

Being aware of such subtleties and conscious of how these foods are incorporated into our diets brings us closer to mastering the art of a renal diet.

2.3. The Role of Fruits and Vegetables

As we continue our journey into the world of the renal diet, we have effortlessly navigated through understanding the significance of sodium, potassium, and phosphorus, as well as selecting healthy protein sources. With a strengthened foundation, we now turn our attention to the enchanting garden of culinary delights: fruits and vegetables.

The Magic of the Garden: Exploring the Benefits of Fruits and Vegetables
Nature's bounty offers a vast selection of fruits and vegetables that can safely fit within the confines of a renal diet. These wondrous foods, aside from their palate-pleasing flavors, serve as fortifying soldiers, supporting our bodies from within. Rich in natural antioxidants, they actively combat inflammation and provide much-needed protection against various chronic diseases.

A renal diet thrives on the natural gifts fruits and vegetables bestow — offering ample dietary fiber that aids in digestion and satiety, balancing blood sugar levels, and maintaining heart health. Simultaneously, their discrete kaleidoscope of nutrients, such as vitamins A, C, K, and B vitamins, all have a robust line-up of essential roles in maintaining overall health and well-being.

Low-Potassium Virtuosos: The Unsung Heroes

Opting for low-potassium fruits and vegetables is paramount for a renal diet, opening doors to a pallet of delightful options. Colorful bell peppers, zucchini, crisp iceberg lettuce, and plump, juicy blueberries and grapes — this is but a glimpse into the realm of low-potassium choices.

Tackling Tautologies: Moderation and Mindfulness

As we journey deeper into the enchanting garden of fruits and vegetables, we occasionally encounter foods that, while captivating, may be high in potassium or other nutrients we need to monitor closely. From tender, meaty avocados to succulent honeydew melons, it isn't about avoiding these foods altogether but rather approaching them with moderation and mindfulness.

Understanding the joy of savoring these precious bites on occasion, rather than indulging in excess, brings balance and harmony to the renal diet.

Phosphorus: A Whisper in the Culinary Symphony

While phosphorus does not make as much noise as potassium in the discussion of renal diet-friendly produce, it too has a small but significant role to play. Certain fruits and vegetables may contain moderately higher levels of phosphorus, such as dried fruits and avocados.

Chapter 3: Mastering the Art of Cooking and Seasoning

3.1. Healthy Cooking Techniques

In the journey of mastering the kidney-friendly cuisine, understanding and implementing various cooking techniques is vital. The tastes, textures, and even the nutritional values of the ingredients can be significantly altered based on the cooking method employed. As you weave your way through the world of the renal diet, grasping these methods will greatly contribute to your kitchen prowess. Let's explore a few examples.

- **Steaming: The Nutrients' Saviour**

Vividly colored and crisp, steamed vegetables are not just visually appealing, but they are a nutrient powerhouse too. While all cooking methods slightly reduce the nutrient content in vegetables, steaming is one method that arguably does the least damage. The indirect heat ensures that the vegetables aren't exposed to scorching temperatures that could destroy heat-sensitive nutrients. The absence of cooking fats in this method makes it an attractive way to manage calories as well.

Also, steaming is not limited to vegetables. It can be used for cooking seafood, poultry, and even certain cuts of meat, rendering them tender, juicy and cooked to perfection—without the need for additional oil or fats.

- **Poaching: Gentle Cooking**

Poaching is a cooking method that uses a liquid, whether it's water, broth or a more creative fluid like wine or tomato sauce, to cook food gently. Because of the gentleness of this method, it's most commonly used for delicate foods like eggs and fish.

Poaching, unlike boiling, isn't at a hot enough temperature to agitate and damage the food. The liquid impart subtle flavors, while the lower temperatures prevent the food from drying out or losing its natural flavors. This method can enable you to create beautifully moist and flavorful dishes, without adding excessive fats or salt.

- **Grilling: Giving Foods a Flavorful Char**

Grilling exposes foods to direct, high heat which creates a slightly charred, smoky exterior while sealing in the natural juices of food. It's not only for summer barbecues, grilling can be done indoors using a stovetop or an electric grill.

The high heat caramelizes the natural sugars in vegetables and fruits, enhancing their flavors. The cooking technique can transform a plain chicken breast into a mouth-watering masterpiece. However, it's essential to limit the charred parts while grilling as those may carry potential health risks.

- **Roasting: Developing Depths of Flavors**

Roasting involves cooking food in an oven at a high temperature. When the heat gently envelops the food, it caramelizes the sugars present in the food, resulting in a deliciously sweet and complex flavor profile. Whether it's winter squashes, tomatoes, bell peppers, or a piece of meat, roasting can coax out an array of flavors.

- **Sautéing: Quick and Effective**

Sautéing is a cooking process that involves cooking food quickly in a small amount of oil or fat. The heat is fairly high, and the food is frequently stirred or tossed to prevent it from burning or sticking to the pan.

Sautéing is excellent for cooking vegetables, making stir-fries, or searing meat. Always be mindful to choose a healthier oil option such as olive oil, and carefully manage the amount to optimize your renal diet.

- **Slow Cooking: Patience Pays Off**

Slow cooking, as the name suggests, involves cooking foods on a lower heat setting for an extended period. It's a wonderful method to infuse flavors deeply into your dishes. Stews, soups, and casseroles are perfect candidates for this cooking method. By letting it slow and steady, you allow the ingredients' flavors to meld together into a harmonious dish that's both comforting and nutritious.

The Art of Technique

Indeed, the cooking technique you opt for can make a significant difference in your renal diet. Not only does it affect the taste and appearance of the food, but it also impacts the nutrients the food delivers. With knowledge of these cooking methods, you are well on your way to become a maestro in the kitchen, one who can conjure up a wholesome and flavorsome meal that honors your kidneys' needs.

3.2. Salt Substitutes and Alternatives

Managing sodium intake is a crucial aspect of a kidney-friendly diet, and finding ways to maintain flavor without relying on traditional table salt is an essential life skill for those looking to cook and season their meals in the healthiest way possible.

The Importance of Limiting Sodium in the Renal Diet

High sodium levels pose a significant risk to those with kidney disease, as kidneys' ability to remove excess sodium is compromised. By opting for salt substitutes and seasoning alternatives, you can successfully harness flavor in your food without compromising your health goals.

Herb and Spice Blends

Countless flavorings can be conjured from the rich world of herbs and spices. Blends of these seasonings can offer a complexity of flavor that rivals and indeed, often surpasses, the tastes that can be obtained from salt alone.

Opting for salt-free blends, ideally homemade, is an excellent way to begin your explorations in this realm. As you gain experience, you can create your mixtures, tailoring each to various dishes and personal preferences.

To get started, consider assembling the following blends:

Italian Blend: Combine oregano, basil, thyme, rosemary, and marjoram for a Mediterranean twist to your meals.

Herbes de Provence: Blend together thyme, basil, rosemary, tarragon, savory, marjoram, oregano, and bay leaves for a trip to the French countryside.

Mexican Blend: Create a spicy and flavorful blend with cumin, chili powder, oregano, garlic powder, onion powder, and paprika.

Umami-rich Ingredients

In addition to herbs and spices, certain ingredients can impart the highly sought-after umami flavor, a savory depth that enhances a dish in a way that salt might traditionally be employed. By incorporating umami-rich ingredients, you give your meals the rich, savory touch they deserve while maintaining kidney-friendly sodium levels.

Notable umami-rich ingredients include:

- **Mushrooms**: The earthy depth of mushrooms provides a strong umami taste that can enhance many dishes, from stir-fries to casseroles.
- **Tomatoes**: Fresh or sundried tomatoes can lend a tangy, savory flavor that enhances many meals, notably pastas, salads, and Mediterranean-themed dishes.
- **Nutritional Yeast**: With its robust, savory taste, nutritional yeast is a popular addition to plant-based meals, imparting a cheesy, umami note that can elevate simple dishes to new heights.

Experiment with these options:

- **Lemon or Lime Juice:** The zesty tang of citrus fruits can add an instant burst of flavor to a myriad of dishes, from salads to grilled meats and fish.
- **Balsamic Vinegar:** With its rich sweetness and acidity, balsamic vinegar can elevate salads, roasted vegetables, and even fruit-based desserts.
- **Apple Cider Vinegar:** Featuring a fruity tang that complements vegetables, grains, and legumes, apple cider vinegar can offer a subtle yet tantalizing touch to your dishes.

3.3. Flavorful Herbs and Spices

Herbs and spices have the power to elevate any dish, adding bursts of color, aroma, and taste to even the simplest of recipes. Below, we delve into a selection of these ingredients, exploring how they can rejuvenate your home cooking and benefit your renal diet.

Basil: The King of Herbs

Basil, with its sweet, peppery taste, and fragrant aroma, has earned its royal title among herbs. An essential ingredient in Mediterranean cuisine, basil works wonders in everything from tomato dishes to pesto sauces. Basil is rich in antioxidants, which can help protect the kidneys from damaging toxins. Use fresh basil — whole leaves or chopped — as a bright addition to salads, pasta dishes, or sandwiches, bringing a burst of flavor to your meals.

Oregano: A Taste of the Mediterranean

Common in Greek and Italian cuisines, oregano imparts a warm, earthy flavor that enlivens meat dishes, herbaceous tomato sauces, and roasted vegetables. This powerful herb possesses antimicrobial characteristics, and its use in a renal diet can contribute to maintaining healthy kidneys. Use dried oregano as a seasoning or fresh leaves for a more pungent taste that transports you to the shores of the Mediterranean.

Cilantro: The Fresh and Lively Option

Cilantro adds a bright, fresh, and citrusy taste to your dishes, making it the perfect addition to salads, salsas, and various Asian and Mexican dishes. As a natural diuretic, cilantro helps the kidneys eliminate excess water and sodium from the body. Don't be shy in utilizing cilantro — finely chopped or torn leaves compliment a variety of dishes, adding flavor without salt.

Turmeric: The Golden Wonder

Turmeric's earthy, warm taste and vibrant golden color have secured its place as a star among spices. Laden with curcumin, an active compound renowned for its antioxidant and anti-inflammatory properties, turmeric can bolster kidney health. Use ground turmeric sparingly to flavor and color rice dishes, soups, or bean curries, unleashing its potential as a culinary and health-enhancing gem.

Ginger: The Invigorating Spice

Ginger offers a zesty, warming flavor that breathes life into a wide array of dishes, from stir-fries and curries to desserts. Ginger's diuretic and anti-inflammatory properties render it a valuable component of renal diets, helping to maintain kidney health. Use fresh, grated ginger or ground ginger to impart its spicy-sweet taste and health benefits.

Rosemary: The Essence of Aroma

Rosemary's fine, needle-like leaves deliver a potent, savory flavor and exhilarating aroma. Often partnered with meat, poultry, and potato dishes, rosemary's antioxidant-rich nature promotes kidney health. Add rosemary sparingly, either fresh or dried, to imbue your dishes with its distinct aroma and rich taste.

Parsley: The Understated Virtuoso

Parsley is known for its bright, herbaceous flavor, often serving as a backdrop to more elaborate dishes. Despite its unassuming nature, parsley is an excellent source of essential nutrients, including vitamin C. Adding parsley — either curly or flat-leaf varieties — to your meal contributes to flavor and kidney health simultaneously. Use it as a garnish, or finely chop the leaves to incorporate them into your dish.

Experiment with different blends and layering techniques. For instance, try rubbing dry spice mixes onto meats, poultry or fish, or create wet rubs by blending herbs and spices with a bit of oil. Experience the beautiful interplay of flavors by finding harmony between complementary culinary notes: a touch of thyme enhances rosemary's depth, while a pinch of cayenne pepper sparks the warmth of cumin.

3.4. Making Homemade Condiments and Dressings

Store-bought condiments and dressings can often be loaded with sodium and hidden additives, but when we make them ourselves, we have full control over the ingredients to ensure that they are kidney-friendly. By crafting our own delectable and health-conscious condiments and dressings, we can elevate our meals while adhering to the guidelines of a renal diet.

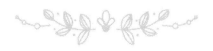

Embracing the World of Homemade Condiments

A well-crafted condiment can enhance the flavors of your dish while staying within the parameters of your kidney-friendly diet. The ingredients we've discussed in the previous sections offer ample opportunities to create homemade condiments brimming with taste and nutrition. Let's explore a few examples of kidney-friendly condiments you can create.

Mustard Magic: Yellow mustard seeds are low in sodium and a versatile base for a healthful condiment. By combining mustard seeds, vinegar, and your choice of herbs and spices, you can make a delightful homemade mustard that accentuates your dishes, adding a punch of flavor without compromising kidney health. Try experimenting with the addition of turmeric, honey, or dill to get a variety of flavors that cater to your taste buds.

Tantalizing Tomato Salsa: Store-bought salsa often contains excessive sodium, but by making your own, you can control the ingredients that go into it. Create a scrumptious and kidney-friendly salsa by combining diced tomatoes, red onion, jalapeño, lime juice, cilantro, and a touch of garlic. The result is a vibrant and zesty salsa perfect for dipping or adding to your favorite dishes.

Savory Soy Alternative: Traditional soy sauce can be surprisingly high in sodium. However, creating a homemade alternative affords you the opportunity to enjoy the umami-rich flavor without the sodium. Combine low-sodium vegetable broth, balsamic vinegar, and a touch of molasses to recreate that savory flavor with significantly less sodium.

Delight Your Palate with Homemade Dressings

A divine dressing can effortlessly elevate a salad or add a burst of flavor to your favorite dish. By making your own dressings using the flavors of herbs and spices, you can create renal-friendly options that meet your nutritional needs and taste preferences.

Lemon Herb Vinaigrette: Citrus can be a delicious alternative to sodium-rich options, and a lemon herb vinaigrette is a perfect example. Combine freshly squeezed lemon juice, extra virgin olive oil, minced garlic, finely chopped fresh herbs (such as basil, oregano, or parsley), and cracked black pepper to create a zesty dressing that awakens your dish.

Creamy Garlic Herb Dressing: A flavorsome dressing does not mean you need to sacrifice creaminess. Blend together plain Greek yogurt, fresh garlic, your choice of fresh herbs (such as dill, basil, or chives), and a splash of lemon juice to create a sumptuous dressing that is both kidney-friendly and satisfying.

Balsamic Berry Vinaigrette: Harness the natural sweetness of berries to create an enticing, fruity dressing for your next salad. Blend fresh or frozen berries (such as strawberries or raspberries), balsamic vinegar, extra virgin olive oil, and a touch of honey or agave syrup to taste. The result is a versatile dressing that combines sweet, tangy, and aromatic flavors that work beautifully with salads, grilled vegetables, or even a fruit salad.

Balance and Creativity: The Key to Successful Homemade Condiments and Dressings
One significant aspect of crafting kidney-friendly condiments and dressings is always striving to achieve balance. To ensure that your homemade creations remain renal diet compliant, pay attention to sodium, potassium, and phosphorus levels and think creatively when adding flavor boosters. Mastering the delicate interplay between tangy, sweet, and spicy flavors will enable you to create condiments and dressings that truly shine without potentially harming kidney health.

Chapter 4: Kickstart Your Morning: Healthy Breakfast Recipes

4.1. Kidney-Friendly Breakfast Smoothies
★ Recipe 1: Morning Zest Smoothie

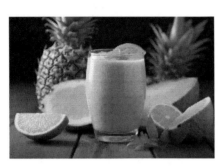

- Preparation Time: 10 minutes

-Serving: 1-2

- Method of Cooking: Blending

Ingredients:

- ½ cup peeled grapefruit,
- 1 ripe peach (pitted),
- ½ cup unsweetened almond milk
- ½ cup pineapple chunks,

Procedure: Blend the grapefruit, pineapple, peach, and unsweetened almond milk together until smooth. Serve immediately.

Nutritional Values (Per Serving): Calories: 154, Fat: 1g, Sodium: 60mg, Carbs: 38g, Fiber: 4g, Protein: 3g

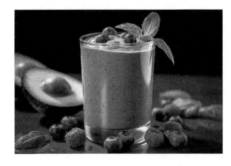

★ Recipe 2: Blueberry Avocado Delight

- Preparation Time: 12 minutes

- Serving: 1-2

- Method of Cooking: Blending

Ingredients:

- ¾ cup blueberries,
- ½ avocado (peeled and pitted),
- 1 cup spinach,
- 1 cup unsweetened almond milk,
- 1 teaspoon honey

Procedure: In a blender, combine the blueberries, avocado, spinach, almond milk, and honey. Blend until smooth and creamy. Serve immediately.

Nutritional Values (Per Serving): Calories: 207, Fat: 10g, Sodium: 54mg, Carbs: 25g, Fiber: 6g, Protein: 4g

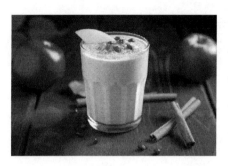

★ Recipe 3: Cinnamon Apple Oats Smoothie

- Preparation Time: 10 minutes

- Serving: 2

- Method of Cooking: Blending

Ingredients:

- 1 medium apple (cored and sliced),
- ¼ cup uncooked rolled oats,
- ½ teaspoon cinnamon,
- 1 ½ cups water

Procedure: Blend the apple, rolled oats, cinnamon, and water until smooth. Serve immediately.

Nutritional Values (Per Serving): Calories: 80, Fat: 1g, Sodium: 2mg, Carbs: 18g, Fiber: 4g, Protein: 2g

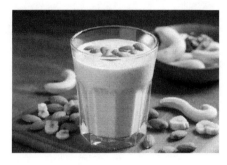

★ Recipe 4: Nourishing Nutty Delight

- Preparation Time: 12 minutes

- Serving: 1-2

- Method of Cooking: Blending

Ingredients:

- ½ cup almond milk,
- 2 tbsp walnut,
- 2 tbsp cashew,
- 1 tbsp flaxseed,
- 1 banana

Procedure: Blend almond milk, walnut, cashew, flaxseed, and peeled banana until a smooth consistency is achieved.

Nutritional Values (Per Serving): Calories: 294, Fat: 22g, Sodium: 15mg, Carbs: 24g, Fiber: 5g, Protein: 10g

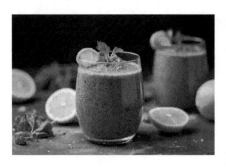

★ Recipe 5: Green Detox Smoothie

- Preparation Time: 10 minutes

- Serving: 1-2

- Method of Cooking: Blending

Ingredients:

- 1 cup kale (chopped),
- 1 cup spinach,
- ½ cucumber,
- ½ peeled lemon,
- 1 cup water

Procedure: Add kale, spinach, cucumber, lemon, and water to a blender. Blend until smooth. Pour into a glass and serve.

Nutritional Values (Per Serving): Calories: 76, Fat: 0.7g, Sodium: 48mg, Carbs: 16g, Fiber: 4g, Protein: 3g

4.2. Low-Sodium Breakfast Delights

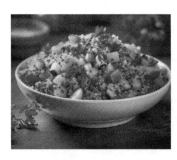

★ Recipe 1: Sunny Quinoa Bowl

- Preparation Time: 20 minutes

- Serving: 2

- Method of Cooking: Boiling and Mixing

Ingredients:

- 1/2 cup uncooked quinoa,
- 1 cup water,
- 1/4 cup chopped bell pepper,
- 1/4 cup diced tomato,
- 1/4 cup diced cucumber,
- 2 tbsp chopped fresh cilantro,
- 1 tbsp olive oil, 1 tbsp lemon juice

Procedure: Cook quinoa according to package instructions. In a large bowl, combine the cooked quinoa, diced vegetables, and fresh cilantro. Drizzle with olive oil and lemon juice, and mix well. Serve at room temperature.

Nutritional Values (Per Serving, in g): Calories: 240, Fat: 9g, Sodium: 30mg, Carbs: 34g, Fiber: 4g, Protein: 8g

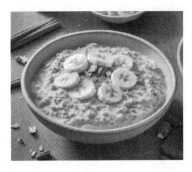

★ Recipe 2: Banana Nut Overnight Oats

- Preparation Time: 10 minutes (+overnight soaking)
- Serving: 2
- Method of Cooking: Mixing

Ingredients:

- 1/2 cup rolled oats,
- 1 cup unsweetened almond milk,
- 1/2 ripe banana (mashed),
- 1 tbsp almond butter,
- 1/4 cup chopped walnuts

Procedure: In a mason jar or container with a lid, mix together oats, almond milk, mashed banana, and almond butter. Stir to combine well. Top with chopped walnuts and place in the fridge overnight. Stir before serving.

Nutritional Values (Per Serving, in g): Calories: 264, Fat: 14g, Sodium: 55mg, Carbs: 30g, Fiber: 5g, Protein: 7g

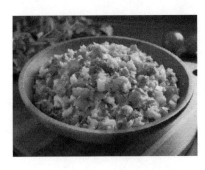

★ Recipe 3: Veggie Egg White Scramble

- Preparation Time: 15 minutes

Serving: 2

Method of Cooking: Sautéing and Scrambling

Ingredients:

- 1/2 cup diced bell pepper,
- 1/2 cup chopped spinach,
- 1/4 cup diced onion,
- 1/4 cup diced tomato,
- 4 egg whites,
- 1 tbsp olive oil,
- black pepper to taste

Procedure: In a non-stick skillet, heat olive oil on medium heat and sauté bell pepper, onion, spinach, and tomato until softened. In a separate bowl, whisk egg whites and pour them over the vegetables. Scramble the mixture until fully cooked. Add black pepper to taste and serve immediately. Nutritional Values (Per Serving, in g): Calories: 125, Fat: 6g, Sodium: 85mg, Carbs: 7g, Fiber: 2g, Protein: 10g

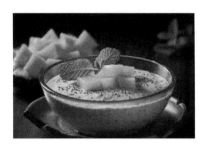

★ Recipe 4: Tropical Chia Pudding

- Preparation Time: 10 minutes (+overnight soaking)

Serving: 2

Method of Cooking: Mixing

Ingredients:

- 1/4 cup chia seeds,
- 1 cup unsweetened coconut milk,
- 1/2 cup diced mango,
- 1/2 cup diced pineapple,
- 1 tbsp honey,
- 1/4 cup unsweetened shredded coconut

Procedure: In a mason jar or container with a lid, combine chia seeds, coconut milk, and honey. Mix well and let it sit for 1-2 minutes, then stir again to prevent clumping. Refrigerate overnight. When ready to serve, top with mango, pineapple, and shredded coconut.

Nutritional Values (Per Serving, in g): Calories: 320, Fat: 18g, Sodium: 25mg, Carbs: 38g, Fiber: 12g, Protein: 6g

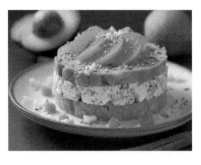

★ Recipe 5: Low-Sodium Rice Cake with Avocado

- Preparation Time: 5 minutes
- Serving: 2
- Method of Cooking: Assembling

Ingredients:

- 2 unsalted rice cakes,
- 1 medium ripe avocado,
- 1 tbsp shredded carrot,
- 1 tbsp finely chopped red onion,

- 1 tsp black pepper,
- 1 tsp crushed red pepper flakes (optional)

Procedure: Slice avocado and place it on top of each rice cake. Divide the shredded carrot and chopped red onion on top of the avocado. Sprinkle black pepper and optional red pepper flakes on top of the assembled rice cakes. Serve immediately.

Nutritional Values (Per Serving, in g): Calories: 163, Fat: 10g, Sodium: 20mg, Carbs: 17g, Fiber: 6g, Protein: 3g

4.3. Plant-based and High-Protein Options

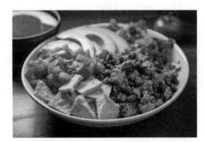

★ Recipe 1: Tofu Scramble

- Preparation Time: 19 minutes

- Serving: 4

- Method of Cooking: Sautéing

Ingredients:

- 1 block of firm tofu,
- 1 cup diced bell peppers,
- 1/2 cup black beans,
- 1/2 cup diced tomatoes,
- 2 tbsp olive oil,
- 1 tbsp nutritional yeast,
- 1 tsp turmeric,
- black pepper to taste

Procedure: Press and crumble tofu into small pieces. In a pan, heat olive oil and sauté the tofu, bell peppers, and black beans. Add in the tomatoes, nutritional yeast, turmeric, and black pepper. Cook until everything is well-mixed and heated through.

Nutritional Values (Per Serving, in g): Calories: 185, Fat: 11g, Sodium: 15mg, Carbs: 10g, Fiber: 4g, Protein: 15g

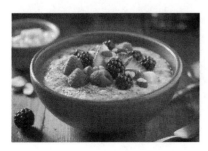

★ **Recipe 2: Vegan Quinoa Porridge**

- Preparation Time: 20 minutes

- Serving: 4

- Method of Cooking: Boiling

Ingredients:

- 1 cup quinoa,
- 2 cups unsweetened almond milk,
- 1 tbsp chia seeds,
- 1/2 cup mixed berries,
- 1 tbsp maple syrup

Procedure: Cook the quinoa according to the package instructions with almond milk instead of water. Once cooked, add chia seeds, mixed berries, and maple syrup. Stir well and cook another 2-3 minutes until heated through.

Nutritional Values (Per Serving, in g): Calories: 218, Fat: 3g, Sodium: 15mg, Carbs: 40g, Fiber: 6g, Protein: 8g

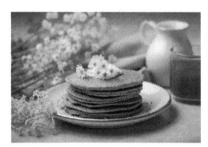

★ **Recipe 3: Buckwheat Pancakes**

- Preparation Time: 30 minutes
- Serving: 4
- Method of Cooking: Frying

Ingredients:

- 1 cup buckwheat flour,
- 1 tbsp flaxseed meal,
- 2 tsp baking powder,
- 1 cup almond milk,
- 1 tbsp sunflower oil,
- fruits for topping

Procedure: Mix the buckwheat flour, flaxseed meal, and baking powder. Add the almond milk and oil to create a batter. Pan fry in a non-stick skillet until golden brown on both sides. Serve topped with fresh fruits.

Nutritional Values (Per Serving, in g): Calories: 158, Fat: 5g, Sodium: 20mg, Carbs: 27g, Fiber: 4g, Protein: 5g

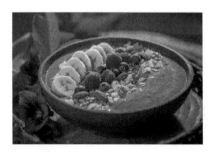

★ **Recipe 4: Chia Berry Smoothie Bowl**

- Preparation Time: 5 minutes
- Serving: 1

- Method of Cooking: Blending

Ingredients:

- 1 banana,
- 1 cup mixed berries,
- 1/2 cup coconut water,
- 2 tbsp chia seeds,
- 1/4 cup granola for topping,
- fresh fruits for topping

Procedure: In a blender, blend banana, mixed berries, coconut water and 1 tbsp of chia seeds until smooth. Pour into a bowl and top with the remaining chia seeds, granola and fresh fruits.

Nutritional Values (Per Serving, in g): Calories: 380, Fat: 10g, Sodium: 60mg, Carbs: 68g, Fiber: 15g, Protein: 9g

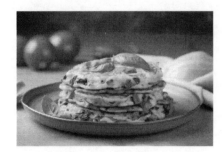

★ Recipe 5: Vegan Chickpea Omelette

- Preparation Time: 15 minutes
- Serving: 1
- Method of Cooking: Sautéing and Frying

Ingredients:

- 1/2 cup chickpea flour,
- 1/2 cup water,
- 1/2 cup vegetables for stuffing (spinach, bell peppers etc),
- 1 tsp olive oil,
- turmeric,
- black pepper to taste

Procedure: Mix the chickpea flour and water to make a batter. In a non-stick skillet, sauté the vegetables with olive oil. Pour batter over the vegetables, cook until golden brown on both sides. Nutritional Values (Per Serving, in g): Calories: 200, Fat: 6g, Sodium: 30mg, Carbs: 30g, Fiber: 6g, Protein: 10g

Chapter 5: Easy and Light Lunches: Stress-free Midday Meals

5.1. Quick and Simple Sandwiches

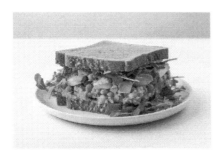

★ Recipe 1: Spicy Avocado and Chickpea Sandwich

- Preparation Time: 15 minutes

- Serving: 2

- Method of Cooking: Mashing and Assembling

Ingredients:

- 1 ripe avocado,
- 1/2 cup canned chickpeas,
- 1 tsp cayenne pepper,
- 1/2 lemon, juiced, salt to taste,
- 4 slices of whole grain bread,
- lettuce and cucumber for topping

Procedure: Mash avocado, chickpeas together in a bowl. Stir in cayenne pepper, lemon juice, and salt. Spread the mixture on slices of bread. Add lettuce and cucumber. Assemble the sandwiches.

Nutritional Values (Per Serving, in g): Calories: 340, Fat: 15g, Sodium: 300mg, Carbs: 45g, Fiber: 15g, Protein: 10g

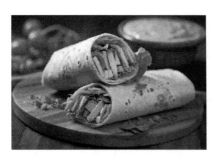

★ **Recipe 2: Veggie Hummus Wrap**

- Preparation Time: 10 minutes

- Serving: 2

- Method of Cooking: Assembling

Ingredients:

- 2 whole grain tortillas,
- 1/2 cup hummus,

- 1 carrot, 1 cucumber,
- 1 bell pepper,
- all thinly sliced

Procedure: Spread hummus on the tortillas. Top with thinly sliced carrot, cucumber, and bell pepper. Roll up the tortillas into a wrap.

Nutritional Values (Per Serving, in g): Calories: 270, Fat: 11g, Sodium: 450mg, Carbs: 31g, Fiber: 10g, Protein: 12g

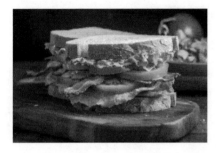

★ Recipe 3: Kidney-Friendly BLT

- Preparation Time: 15 minutes

- Serving: 2

- Method of Cooking: Frying and Assembling

Ingredients:

- 4 slices of low sodium bacon,
- 4 slices of whole grain bread,
- 2 large lettuce leaves,
- 2 tomato slices,
- 2 tbsp low-fat mayonnaise

Procedure: Cook the bacon until crispy. Spread mayonnaise on the bread slices. Layer bacon, lettuce, and tomato onto two slices and close the sandwiches with the remaining slices.

Nutritional Values (Per Serving, in g): Calories: 275, Fat: 10g, Sodium: 325mg, Carbs: 30g, Fiber: 5g, Protein: 15g

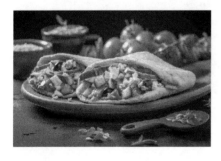

★ Recipe 4: Mediterranean Veggie Pita

- Preparation Time: 15 minutes

- Serving: 2

- Method of Cooking: Assembling

Ingredients:

- 2 whole grain pitas,
- 1/2 cup hummus,

- 1/2 cup chopped cucumber,
- 1/2 cup diced tomatoes,
- 1/4 cup sliced olives,
- 1/4 cup crumbled feta

Procedure: Slice the pitas open to create a pocket. Spread hummus inside each one. Fill with cucumber, tomatoes, olives, and feta.

Nutritional Values (Per Serving, in g): Calories: 320, Fat: 12g, Sodium: 540mg, Carbs: 42g, Fiber: 8g, Protein: 12g

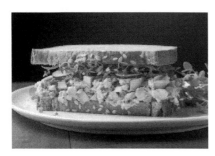

★ **Recipe 5: Tofu Salad Sandwich**

- Preparation Time: 15 minutes

- Serving: 2

- Method of Cooking: Mixing and Assembling

Ingredients:

- 8 oz firm tofu,
- 2 tbsp low-fat mayonnaise,
- 1/2 red onion, diced,
- 1/2 celery stalk,
- chopped,
- black pepper to taste,
- 4 slices of whole grain bread,
- lettuce and tomato for topping

Procedure: Combine crumbled tofu, mayonnaise, red onion, and celery. Season with pepper. Spread the mixture onto bread slices. Add lettuce and tomato, then close sandwiches with remaining slices.

Nutritional Values (Per Serving, in g): Calories: 275, Fat: 10g, Sodium: 325mg, Carbs: 30g, Fiber: 5g, Protein: 15g

5.2. Delightful Salads

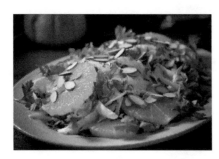

★ Recipe 1: Tangy Citrus and Fennel Salad

- Preparation Time: 15 minutes

- Serving: 2

- Method of Cooking: Tossing

Ingredients:

- 2 cups mixed salad greens,
- 1 fennel bulb, thinly sliced,
- 1 orange, peeled and sectioned,
- 1/4 cup sliced almonds,

- 1 tbsp olive oil,
- 1 tbsp lemon juice,
- salt and black pepper to taste

Procedure: In a large bowl, toss salad greens, fennel, orange, and almonds. Drizzle with olive oil, lemon juice, salt, and pepper. Toss to combine.

Nutritional Values (Per Serving, in g): Calories: 210, Fat: 12g, Sodium: 110mg, Carbs: 25g, Fiber: 7g, Protein: 5g

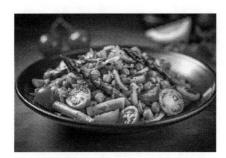

★ Recipe 2: Grilled Asparagus and Chickpea Salad

- Preparation Time: 20 minutes

- Serving: 2

- Method of Cooking: Tossing

Ingredients:

- 1 cup grilled asparagus, chopped,
- 1/2 cup canned chickpeas,
- 1/2 cup cherry tomatoes,
- halved,

- 1/4 cup diced red onion,
- 1 tbsp olive oil,
- 1 tbsp apple cider vinegar,
- salt and black pepper to taste

Procedure: Combine grilled asparagus, chickpeas, tomatoes, and red onion in a bowl. Mix with olive oil, vinegar, salt, and pepper.

Nutritional Values (Per Serving, in g): Calories: 225, Fat: 8g, Sodium: 215mg, Carbs: 30g, Fiber: 9g, Protein: 8g

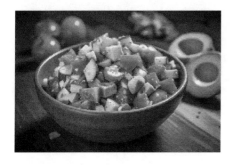

★ Recipe 3: Cucumber, Tomato, and Avocado Salad

- Preparation Time: 10 minutes

- Serving: 2

- Method of Cooking: Tossing

Ingredients:

- 1 cucumber, diced,
- 1 tomato, diced,
- 1 ripe avocado,
- diced,
- 1/4 cup chopped fresh parsley,
- 2 tbsp lemon juice,
- olive oil,
- salt and black pepper to taste

Procedure: Toss cucumber, tomato, avocado, and parsley in a bowl. Stir in lemon juice, olive oil, salt, and pepper. Nutritional Values (Per Serving, in g): Calories: 255, Fat: 20g, Sodium: 15mg, Carbs: 20g, Fiber: 8g, Protein: 3g

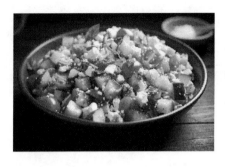

★ Recipe 4: Greek Quinoa Salad

- Preparation Time: 25 minutes

- Serving: 2

- Method of Cooking: Tossing

Ingredients:

- 1 cup cooked quinoa,
- 1/2 cup diced cucumber,
- 1/2 cup diced tomatoes,
- 1/4 cup sliced olives,

- 1/4 cup crumbled feta,
- 2 tbsp olive oil,
- 1 tbsp lemon juice,
- fresh parsley

Procedure: Combine quinoa, cucumber, tomatoes, olives, and feta in a bowl. Dress with olive oil and lemon juice. Garnish with parsley. Nutritional Values (Per Serving, in g): Calories: 385, Fat: 21g, Sodium: 530mg, Carbs: 40g, Fiber: 5g, Protein: 12g

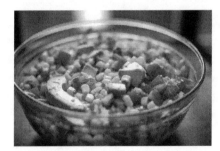

★ Recipe 5: Summer Corn and Avocado Salad

- Preparation Time: 15 minutes

- Serving: 2

- Method of Cooking: Tossing

Ingredients:

- 1 cup fresh corn kernels,
- 1 ripe avocado, diced,
- 1 red bell pepper, diced,
- 1/4 cup chopped fresh cilantro,

- 2 tbsp lime juice,
- olive oil,
- salt and black pepper to taste

Procedure: Toss corn kernels, avocado, red bell pepper, and cilantro in a bowl. Stir in lime juice, olive oil, salt, and pepper.Nutritional Values (Per Serving, in g): Calories: 245, Fat: 15g, Sodium: 15mg, Carbs: 29g, Fiber: 8g, Protein: 4g

5.3. Hearty and Healthy Soups

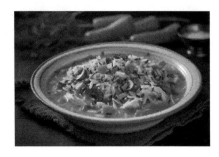 ★ Recipe 1: Chicken and Wild Rice Soup

- Preparation Time: 1 hour

- Serving: 2

- Method of Cooking: Simmering

Ingredients:

- 1 cup cubed chicken breasts,
- 1 cup cooked wild rice,
- 1/2 cup diced carrots,
- 1/2 cup diced celery,
- 1/4 cup diced onion,
- 1 clove garlic,
- minced,
- 4 cups low-sodium chicken broth,
- 1/2 tsp dried thyme,
- olive oil,
- salt and black pepper to taste

Procedure: In a pot, sauté chicken, onions, and garlic in olive oil. Add carrots, celery, thyme, salt, and black pepper. Pour in the broth and bring to a simmer, stirring occasionally. Add the cooked wild rice and simmer for another 20 minutes.

Nutritional Values (Per Serving, in g): Calories: 290, Fat: 8g, Sodium: 530mg, Carbs: 30g, Fiber: 4g, Protein: 25g

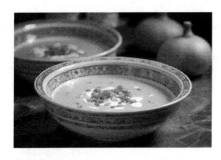

★ Recipe 2: Creamy Butternut Squash Soup

- Preparation Time: 45 minutes

- Serving: 2

- Method of Cooking: Simmering

Ingredients:

- 2 cups cubed butternut squash,
- 1/2 cup diced onion,
- 1 clove garlic, minced,
- 2 cups vegetable broth,

- 1/4 cup low-fat milk,
- olive oil,
- salt and black pepper to taste

Procedure: In a pot, sauté onions and garlic in olive oil. Add butternut squash, salt, and black pepper. Pour in the broth and simmer until butternut is soft. Blend the soup until smooth, then return to the pot. Stir in the milk and cook for another 5 minutes.

Nutritional Values (Per Serving, in g): Calories: 230, Fat: 9g, Sodium: 530mg, Carbs: 35g, Fiber: 6g, Protein: 5g

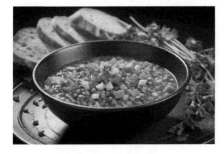

★ Recipe 3: Lentil and Vegetable Soup

- Preparation Time: 40 minutes

- Serving: 2

- Method of Cooking: Boiling

Ingredients:

- 1/2 cup lentils,
- 1/2 cup diced carrot,
- 1/2 cup diced celery,
- 1/2 cup diced tomatoes,

- 4 cups vegetable broth,
- 1 clove garlic, minced,
- olive oil,
- salt and black pepper to taste

Procedure: In a pot, sauté garlic in olive oil. Add carrot, celery, tomatoes, lentils, salt, and black pepper. Pour in the broth and bring to a boil. Reduce heat and simmer until lentils and vegetables are tender.

Nutritional Values (Per Serving, in g): Calories: 180, Fat: 3g, Sodium: 530mg, Carbs: 30g, Fiber: 7g, Protein: 12g

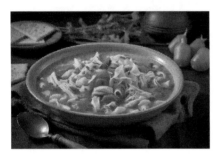

★ Recipe 4: Chicken Noodle Soup

- Preparation Time: 30 minutes

- Serving: 2

- Method of Cooking: Boiling

Ingredients:

- 1 cup cubed chicken breasts,
- 1/2 cup uncooked whole wheat noodles,
- 1/2 cup diced carrots,
- 1/2 cup diced celery,
- 4 cups low-sodium chicken broth,
- 1 clove garlic, minced,
- olive oil,
- salt and black pepper to taste

Procedure: In a pot, sauté chicken and garlic in olive oil. Add carrots and celery, stirring occasionally. Pour in the broth, bring to a boil, then add the noodles. Cook until noodles are done and vegetables are tender.

Nutritional Values (Per Serving, in g): Calories: 240, Fat: 5g, Sodium: 530mg, Carbs: 25g, Fiber: 4g, Protein: 25g

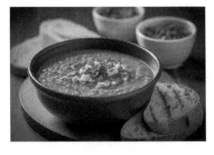

★ Recipe 5: Red Lentil and Sweet Potato Soup

- Preparation Time: 30 minutes

- Serving: 2

- Method of Cooking: Simmering

Ingredients:

- 1/2 cup red lentils,
- 1 large sweet potato (cubed),

- 4 cups low-sodium vegetable broth,
- 1 small onion (chopped),
- 2 cloves garlic (minced),
- 1 teaspoon fresh ginger (grated),
- 1/2 teaspoon ground cumin,
- 2 tablespoons olive oil,
- salt and black pepper to taste

Procedure: Heat the olive oil in a pot and sauté the onion, garlic, ginger, and cumin until fragrant. Add the red lentils, sweet potato, salt, and black pepper. Stir everything together before pouring in the vegetable broth. Bring to a simmer, cover, and cook for about 40 minutes until the lentils and sweet potato are tender. If you prefer a smoother texture, use a hand blender to puree the soup.

Nutritional Values (Per Serving, in g): Calories: 315, Fat: 6g, Sodium: 530mg, Carbs: 48g, Fiber: 15g, Protein: 14g

Chapter 6: Indulge your Palate: Gourmet Lunch Recipes

6.1. Elegant Seafood Options

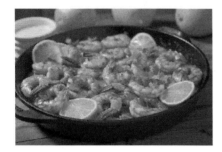

★ Recipe 1: Grilled Shrimp with Rosemary Lemon Sauce

- Preparation Time: 25 minutes

- Serving: 2

- Method of Cooking: Grilling

Ingredients:

- 12 medium-size shrimps,
- peeled and deveined,
- 2 lemons (juiced),
- 2 cloves of garlic minced,

- 1 tablespoon of fresh rosemary (chopped),
- 2 tablespoons of olive oil,
- black pepper to taste

Procedure: Marinate the shrimp in a mixture of lemon juice, garlic, rosemary, olive oil, and black pepper for 20 minutes. Preheat a grill on medium heat and grill shrimp on each side for 3 minutes until opaque and pink.

Nutritional Values (Per Serving, in g): Calories: 170, Fat: 8g, Sodium: 135mg, Carbs: 3g, Fiber: 0g, Protein: 23g

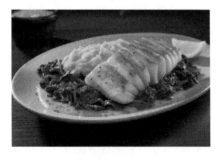

★ Recipe 2: Pan-Seared Cod with Sautéed Spinach

- Preparation Time: 30 minutes

- Serving: 2

- Method of Cooking: Pan Searing

Ingredients:

- 2 cod fillets,
- 2 cups of fresh spinach,
- 2 cloves of garlic (minced),

- 1/2 tbsp chili flakes,
- 2 tablespoons of oil,
- salt and black pepper to taste

Procedure: Season the cod with salt, and pepper. Heat oil in a pan and sear the cod for 5 minutes on each side. In the same pan, sauté garlic and chili flakes until fragrant. Add the spinach and cook until wilted. Serve the cod over a bed of sautéed spinach.

Nutritional Values (Per Serving, in g): Calories: 240, Fat: 9g, Sodium: 80mg, Carbs: 1g, Fiber: 1g, Protein: 35g

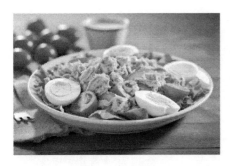

★ **Recipe 3: Tuna Nicoise Salad**

- Preparation Time: 25 minutes

- Serving: 2

- Method of Cooking: No Cook

Ingredients:

- 100g canned low-sodium Tuna (drained),
- 2 medium-sized boiled eggs,
- 2 handfuls of mixed salad greens,
- 10 cherry tomatoes (halved),
- 1/4 cucumber (sliced),

- 10 black olives (pitted),
- dressing: 1 tbsp olive oil,
- 1 tsp Dijon mustard,
- 1 tbsp white wine vinegar, black pepper to taste.

Procedure: Toss together salad greens, cherry tomatoes, cucumber and black olives in a serving bowl. Scatter drained tuna over salad. Cut the boiled eggs into quarters and arrange them around the bowl. Whisk together olive oil, mustard, vinegar, and black pepper to make the dressing. Drizzle the dressing over the salad before serving.

Nutritional Values (Per Serving, in g): Calories: 300, Fat: 15g, Sodium: 270mg, Carbs: 10g, Fiber: 3g, Protein: 30g

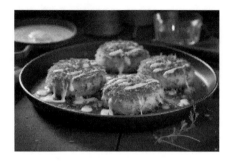

★ Recipe 4: Easy Crab Cakes

- Preparation Time: 30 minutes

- Serving: 2-3

- Method of Cooking: Pan-Frying

Ingredients:

- 4 50g crab meat, 1 tbsp Dijon mustard,
- 1/4 cup breadcrumb,
- 1 egg (lightly beaten),
- 1 tbsp fresh parsley (chopped),
- 1/2 teaspoon Old Bay seasoning,
- 2 tbsp olive oil

Procedure: Combine together crab meat, Dijon mustard, breadcrumb, lightly beaten egg, chopped parsley, and Old Bay seasoning in a bowl. Form 4-6 patties with the mixture. Heat oil in a pan over medium heat and fry the crab cakes for 5 minutes each side or until golden brown.

Nutritional Values (Per Serving, in g): Calories: 210, Fat: 6g, Sodium: 470mg, Carbs: 5g, Fiber: 1g, Protein: 32g

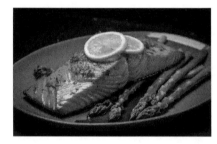

★ Recipe 5: Poached Salmon with Asparagus

- Preparation Time: 30 minutes

- Serving: 2

- Method of Cooking: Poaching

Ingredients:

- 2 salmon fillets,
- 1 bunch of asparagus (trimmed),
- 1 cup of white wine,
- 1 cup of water,
- 1 lemon,
- 1 tbsp olive oil,
- salt and black pepper to taste

Procedure: In a pot, combine white wine, water, juice from one lemon, and a pinch of salt. Bring to a simmer and add salmon fillets. Poach for about 8 minutes until salmon is cooked through. In a separate pan, sauté asparagus in olive oil seasoned with black pepper until tender but still slightly crispy. Serve the poached salmon alongside sautéed asparagus.

Nutritional Values (Per Serving, in g): Calories: 330, Fat: 15g, Sodium: 170mg, Carbs: 5g, Fiber: 2g, Protein: 33g

6.2. Delectable Meat Dishes

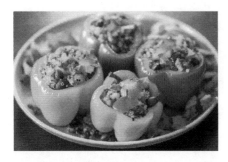

★ Recipe 1: Quinoa Stuffed Bell Peppers

- Preparation Time: 45 minutes

- Serving: 4

- Method of Cooking: Baking

Ingredients:

- 4 bell peppers,
- 1 cup cooked quinoa,
- 1 can black beans (rinsed and drained),
- 1/2 cup corn,
- 1/2 cup chopped onion,
- 2 garlic cloves (minced),
- 1 tsp cumin,
- 1/2 tsp chili powder,
- olive oil,
- salt and pepper to taste

Procedure: Preheat oven to 350°F (175°C). Cut off the tops of bell peppers and remove seeds. In a pan, sauté onion and garlic in olive oil until fragrant, then add black beans, corn, cumin, chili powder, quinoa, and season with salt and pepper. Fill the bell peppers with the quinoa mixture and place them on a baking tray. Bake for about 30 minutes until bell peppers are tender.

Nutritional Values (Per Serving, in g): Calories: 200, Fat: 5g, Sodium: 220mg, Carbs: 34g, Fiber: 7g, Protein: 8g

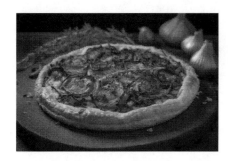

★ Recipe 2: Caramelized Onion and Mushroom Tart

- Preparation Time: 1 hour

- Serving: 4

- Method of Cooking: Baking

Ingredients:

- 1 pre-made pastry shell,
- 2 large onions (sliced),
- 200g mushrooms (sliced),
- 2 tbsp olive oil,

- 1/4 cup white wine,
- 2 tbsp balsamic vinegar,
- 1 tbsp thyme leaves,
- salt and pepper to taste

Procedure: Preheat the oven to 400°F (200°C) and bake the pastry shell according to its package instructions. Meanwhile, heat the olive oil in a pan and add onions, cook till they start to caramelize. Add the mushrooms, white wine, balsamic vinegar, thyme, salt, and pepper. Cook for a further 10 minutes until the mushrooms are soft. Once the pastry shell is ready and cooled, fill it with the onion and mushroom mixture. Place the tart back in the oven for about 10 minutes until it is heated through.

Nutritional Values (Per Serving, in g): Calories: 310, Fat: 18g, Sodium: 160mg, Carbs: 32g, Fiber: 2g, Protein: 5g

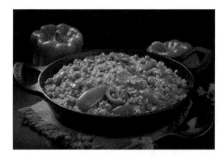

★ **Recipe 3: Vegetable Paella with Saffron**

- Preparation Time: 1 hour

- Serving: 4

- Method of Cooking: Simmering

Ingredients:

- 1 cup Arborio rice, 1 onion (chopped),
- 1 bell pepper (diced),
- 1 cup green peas,
- 2 cloves garlic (minced),

- 3 cups vegetable broth,
- 1 tsp saffron threads,
- 1/2 tsp smoked paprika,
- 2 tbsp olive oil,
- salt and pepper to taste

Procedure: Heat olive oil in a paella pan or large skillet. Add onion and bell pepper, sauté until softened. Add garlic, saffron, and smoked paprika. Stir in the Arborio rice and cook for a couple of minutes until slightly toasted. Pour in vegetable broth and bring to a boil. Reduce heat to low, cover, and simmer for about 20 minutes, stirring occasionally, until rice is tender. Stir in the peas and season with salt and pepper.

Nutritional Values (Per Serving, in g): Calories: 310, Fat: 8g, Sodium: 300mg, Carbs: 54g, Fiber: 4g, Protein: 7g

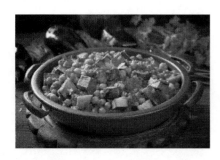

★ Recipe 4: Eggplant and Chickpea Stew

- Preparation Time: 45 minutes

- Serving: 4

- Method of Cooking: Simmering

Ingredients:

- 2 medium eggplants (cubed),
- 1 can chickpeas (rinsed and drained),
- 1 onion (chopped),
- 2 cloves garlic (minced),
- 1 can diced tomatoes,

- 1/2 tsp ground cumin,
- 1/4 tsp ground coriander,
- 1/4 tsp smoked paprika,
- 2 tbsp olive oil,
- salt and pepper to taste

Procedure: In a large pot, heat olive oil and sauté onion and garlic until fragrant. Add eggplant cubes and cook for about 5 minutes until they begin to soften. Stir in chickpeas, diced tomatoes, cumin, coriander, smoked paprika, salt, and pepper. Simmer stew for 20-25 minutes until eggplant is tender. Serve with rice or crusty bread. Nutritional Values (Per Serving, in g): Calories: 310, Fat: 11g, Sodium: 250mg, Carbs: 46g, Fiber: 12g, Protein: 11g

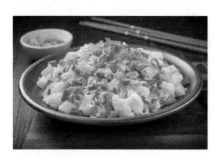

★ Recipe 5: Cauliflower Fried "Rice"

- Preparation Time: 30 minutes

- Serving: 4

- Method of Cooking: Sautéing

Ingredients:

- 1 large cauliflower head (grated or processed into rice-like grains),
- 1 cup of mixed vegetables (such as carrots, peas, and corn),
- 1 onion (chopped),
- 2 cloves of garlic (minced),
- 2 tbsp soy sauce (low sodium),
- 1 tbsp sesame oil,
- salt, and pepper to taste

Procedure: In a large non-stick skillet, heat sesame oil and sauté onion and garlic until golden. Add mixed vegetables, cook until tender. Add cauliflower "rice" and soy sauce, cook for about 5 minutes, stirring occasionally until heated through. Season with salt and pepper to taste. Serve hot as a side dish or a main course.

Nutritional Values (Per Serving, in g): Calories: 145, Fat: 5g, Sodium: 240mg, Carbs: 20g, Fiber: 6g, Protein: 6g

Chapter 7: Light Dinners: Ending the Day on a Healthy Note

7.1. Energy-Boosting Meat Dishes

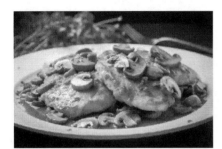

★ Recipe 1: Chicken Marsala with Sautéed Mushrooms

- Preparation Time: 45 minutes

- Serving: 2

- Method of Cooking: Sautéing

Ingredients:

- 2 boneless, skinless chicken breasts,
- 1 cup sliced mushrooms,
- 1/2 cup Marsala wine,

- 2 tbsp olive oil,
- 2 tbsp cornstarch,
- salt and black pepper to taste

Procedure: Season chicken breasts with salt and black pepper on both sides. In a large skillet over medium heat, heat olive oil and sear chicken until golden brown on both sides, then remove from the skillet. Add mushrooms to the same skillet, sauté until softened. Add Marsala wine and scrape the pan to remove any stuck bits. Lower the heat and return chicken to the skillet, simmering in the Marsala and mushroom sauce for around 10 minutes or until chicken is thoroughly cooked. You can thicken the sauce with cornstarch if needed.

Nutritional Values (Per Serving, in g): Calories: 370, Fat: 15g, Sodium: 135mg, Carbs: 12g, Fiber: 1g, Protein: 40g

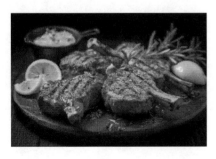

★ **Recipe 2: Grilled Lemon-Thyme Lamb Chops**

- Preparation Time: 35 minutes

- Serving: 2

- Method of Cooking: Grilling

Ingredients:

- 4 lamb chops,
- juice of 2 lemons,
- 2 tbsp fresh thyme leaves (chopped),
- 2 tbsp olive oil,
- salt and black pepper to taste

Procedure: Marinate the lamb chops with lemon juice, olive oil, thyme, salt, and black pepper. Allow it to sit for at least 15 minutes. Heat the grill over high heat. Grill the lamb chops for around 4-5 minutes on each side or until they reach your desired level of doneness.

Nutritional Values (Per Serving, in g): Calories: 375, Fat: 27g, Sodium: 85mg, Carbs: 2g, Fiber: 1g, Protein: 29g

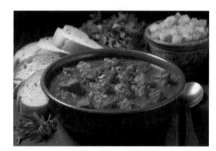

★ **Recipe 3: Italian-Style Beef Ragu**

- Preparation Time: 2 houres

- Serving: 4

- Method of Cooking: Slow-cooking

Ingredients:

- 1 lb beef stew meat,
- 2 cups tomato sauce,
- 1 onion (chopped),
- 3 cloves garlic (minced),
- 2 tbsp olive oil,
- 1 tsp dried basil,
- 1 tsp dried oregano,
- salt and black pepper to taste

Procedure: In a large pot, heat the olive oil over medium heat. Add the chopped onion and minced garlic, sautéing until the onion turns translucent. Add the beef stew meat and brown on all sides. Once the meat is browned, add the tomato sauce, basil, oregano, salt, and black pepper. Stir everything to combine, then lower the heat, cover the pot, and let it simmer for about 2 hours until the meat is tender and the flavors are well combined.

Nutritional Values (Per Serving, in g): Calories: 410, Fat: 20g, Sodium: 365mg, Carbs: 11g, Fiber: 3g, Protein: 48g

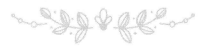

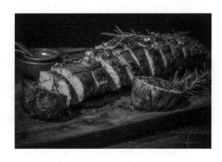 **★ Recipe 4: Roasted Pork Tenderloin with Rosemary and Garlic**

- Preparation Time: 50 minutes

- Serving: 2

- Method of Cooking: Roasting

Ingredients:

- 1 lb pork tenderloin,
- 4 cloves garlic (minced),
- 2 tbsp fresh rosemary leaves (minced),
- 2 tbsp olive oil,
- salt and black pepper to taste

Procedure: Preheat oven to 375°F (190°C). In a small bowl, mix minced garlic, rosemary, olive oil, salt, and black pepper. Rub this mixture all over the pork tenderloin. Place the tenderloin in a roasting pan and bake for about 30 minutes until the internal temperature reaches 145-160°F (63-71°C). Let it rest for a few minutes before slicing.

Nutritional Values (Per Serving, in g): Calories: 410, Fat: 15g, Sodium: 90mg, Carbs: 3g, Fiber: 1g, Protein: 60g

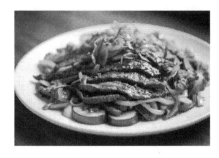

★ **Recipe 5: Tangy Balsamic Steak Stir-Fry**

- Preparation Time: 40 minutes

- Serving: 2

- Method of Cooking: Stir-frying

Ingredients:

- 1 lb lean steak (cut into thin strips),
- 1 bell pepper (julienned),
- 1 zucchini (julienned),

- 1/2 cup balsamic vinegar,
- 2 tbsp olive oil,
- salt and black pepper to taste

Procedure: In a large skillet or wok, heat 1 tablespoon of olive oil over high heat. Quickly stir-fry the steak strips for approximately 2-3 minutes, then remove them and set aside. In the same skillet, add the remaining 1 tablespoon of oil and stir-fry the vegetables until they're tender but still retain some crispness. Return the steak to the skillet, and add the balsamic vinegar, simmering for a few minutes until the sauce thickens and coats all ingredients. Season with salt and black pepper to taste.

Nutritional Values (Per Serving, in g): Calories: 400, Fat: 20g, Sodium: 110mg, Carbs: 18g, Fiber: 4g, Protein: 38g

7.2. Fresh and Flavorful Seafood Recipes

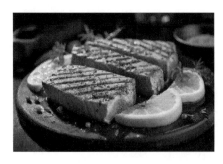

★ Recipe 1: Grilled Tuna Steaks with Citrus Glaze

- Preparation Time: 30 minutes

- Serving: 2

- Method of Cooking: Grilling

Ingredients:

- 2
tuna steaks
- Juice and zest of 1 orange

- Juice and zest of 1 lemon
- 2 tbsp olive oil
- Salt and black pepper to taste

Procedure: In a bowl, combine the orange and lemon juices, their zest, olive oil, salt, and pepper to make a marinade. Marinate the tuna steaks for at least 15 minutes. Preheat a grill and cook the tuna steaks for about 4-5 minutes per side. Be sure not to overcook as tuna can dry out quickly.

Nutritional Values (Per Serving, in g): Calories: 395, Fat: 15g, Sodium: 75mg, Carbs: 9g, Fiber: 1g, Protein: 56g

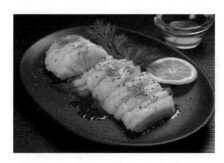

★ Recipe 2: Lemon and Dill Baked Cod

- Preparation Time: 35 minutes

- Serving: 2

- Method of Cooking: Baking

Ingredients:

- 2 cod fillets
- Juice of 1 lemon
- 2 tbsp fresh dill (chopped)
- 2 tbsp olive oil
- Salt and black pepper to taste

Procedure: Preheat oven to 375°F (190°C). Arrange the cod fillets on a baking sheet, drizzle with olive oil, and sprinkle with salt and pepper. Squeeze lemon juice over the top and sprinkle with chopped dill. Bake for 20-25 minutes, or until fish is flaky and opaque. Nutritional Values (Per Serving, in g): Calories: 265, Fat: 13g, Sodium: 95mg, Carbs: 3g, Fiber: 1g, Protein: 32g

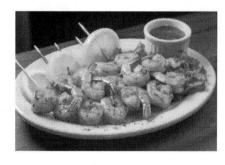

★ Recipe 3: Garlic Butter Shrimp Skewers

- Preparation Time: 30 minutes

- Serving: 2

- Method of Cooking: Grilling

Ingredients:

- 1 lb shrimp (peeled and deveined)
- 4 cloves garlic (minced)
- 2 tbsp butter (melted)

- 1 tbsp fresh parsley (chopped)
- Salt and black pepper to taste

Procedure: Skewer the shrimp onto wooden or metal skewers. In a bowl, mix the minced garlic with the melted butter, then brush this mixture onto the shrimp skewers. Season them with salt and pepper. Grill the skewers for about 2-3 minutes on each side, or until shrimp are pink and opaque. Garnish with chopped parsley before serving.

Nutritional Values (Per Serving, in g): Calories: 365, Fat: 16g, Sodium: 295mg, Carbs: 5g, Fiber: 0g, Protein: 50g

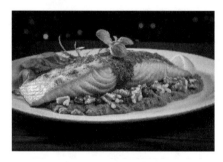

★ Recipe 4: Baked Salmon with Spinach Pesto

- Preparation Time: 40 minutes

- Serving: 2

- Method of Cooking: Baking

Ingredients:

- 2 salmon fillets
- 2 cups fresh spinach
- 1/2 cup fresh basil
- 1/4 cup walnuts

- 1/4 cup olive oil
- 2 cloves garlic
- Salt and pepper to taste

Procedure: Preheat the oven to 375°F (190°C). In a food processor, combine spinach, basil, walnuts, garlic, olive oil, salt, and pepper to create the pesto. Arrange the salmon fillets in a baking dish and spread a generous amount of pesto on each. Bake for 15-20 minutes, or until salmon is cooked to your liking.

Nutritional Values (Per Serving, in g): Calories: 420, Fat: 31g, Sodium: 125mg, Carbs: 7g, Fiber: 3g, Protein: 30g

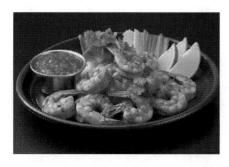

★ Recipe 5: Sweet Chili Lime Grilled Shrimp

- Preparation Time: 30 minutes

- Serving: 2

- Method of Cooking: Grilling

Ingredients:

- 1 lb shrimp (peeled and deveined)
- Juice and zest of 1 lime
- 2 tbsp sweet chili sauce
- 1 tsp soy sauce (low sodium)
- 1 tbsp olive oil

Procedure: In a marinating dish, combine the lime juice, lime zest, sweet chili sauce, and soy sauce. Add the shrimp and let them marinate for at least 15 minutes. Preheat a grill and cook the shrimp for 2-3 minutes on each side, brushing them with marinade as they cook. Shrimp should be pink and opaque when fully cooked.

Nutritional Values (Per Serving, in g): Calories: 320, Fat: 10g, Sodium: 350mg, Carbs: 15g, Fiber: 0g, Protein: 40g

7.3. Plant-Based Delights for Vegetarians and Vegans

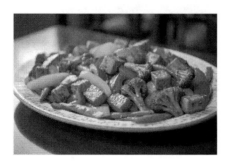

★ Recipe 1: Veggie Tofu Stir–fry

- Preparation Time: 30 minutes

- Serving: 2

- Method of Cooking: Stir-frying

Ingredients:

- 1 block firm tofu
- 1 bell pepper (sliced)
- 1 cup broccoli florets
- 1 cup snap peas
- 2 tbsp low-sodium soy sauce (or tamari)

- 2 tbsp sesame oil
- 1 tsp ginger (minced)
- 2 cloves garlic (minced)
- Servings: 2

Procedure:

Press tofu for 15 minutes to remove excess water then cube it.

In a large pan or wok, heat the sesame oil. Add the tofu, stirring occasionally until it is browned on all sides. Remove from pan and set aside.

In the same pan, add additional oil if necessary, then add the sliced pepper, broccoli, and snap peas. Cook until the vegetables are tender-crisp.

Add back the tofu along with the garlic, ginger, and soy sauce. Stir all ingredients together and cook for another 5 minutes, until everything is hot and well mixed.

Nutritional values (Per Serving, in g): Calories: 275, Fat: 12g, Sodium: 300mg, Carbs: 18g, Fiber: 4g, Protein: 24g

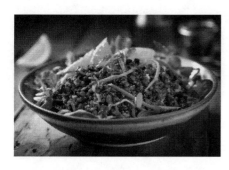

★ Recipe 2: Quinoa and Lentil Salad

- Preparation Time: 25 minutes

- Serving: 2

- Method of Cooking: Boiling

Ingredients:

- 1/2 cup quinoa
- 1/2 cup lentils
- 2 cups vegetable broth (low-sodium)
- 1 cup mixed salad greens

- 1 medium carrot (grated)
- 2 tbsp olive oil
- Juice of 1 lemon

Procedure:

Combine quinoa and vegetable broth in a pot and bring to a boil. Once boiling, reduce heat and simmer until quinoa is soft and has absorbed the broth. Repeat the same process for lentils in a separate pot.

Mix together cooked quinoa and lentils, then let cool.

Once cooled, add in the salad greens and grated carrot.

Dress the salad with olive oil and lemon juice.

Nutritional values (Per serving, in g): Calories: 350, Fat: 14g, Sodium: 180mg, Carbs: 45g, Fiber: 13g, Protein: 15g

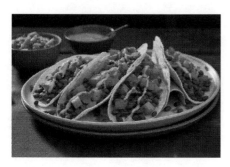

★ Recipe 3: Baked Sweet Potato and Black Bean Tacos

- Preparation Time: 40 minutes

- Serving: 2

- Method of Cooking: Baking

Ingredients:

- 2 medium sweet potatoes
- 1 can low-sodium black beans
- 1 red onion (sliced)
- 1 tbsp olive oil

- 1 tsp cumin
- 1/2 tsp chili powder
- 4 small tortillas

Procedure:

Preheat the oven to 400°F (200°C). Dice the sweet potatoes into small pieces and spread them out on a baking sheet. In a bowl, toss the sweet potatoes with olive oil, cumin, and chili powder.

Bake sweet potatoes for 20-25 minutes or until they are soft.

Once done, assemble the tacos by placing some of the sweet potato in each tortilla, top with black beans and sliced red onion.

Nutritional values (Per serving, in g): Calories: 230, Fat: 5g, Sodium: 500mg, Carbs: 40g, Fiber: 10g, Protein: 8g

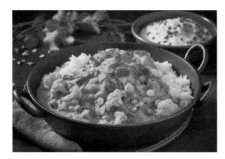

★ Recipe 4: Roasted Cauliflower and Chickpea Curry

- Preparation Time: 45 minutes
- Serving: 4
- Method of Cooking: Roasting

Ingredients:

- 1 head cauliflower (cut into florets)
- 1 can chickpeas (low-sodium)
- 1 cup coconut milk

- 2 tbsp curry powder
- 1 tbsp olive oil
- Salt to taste

Procedure:

Preheat the oven to 425°F (220°C). Toss the cauliflower florets in olive oil and curry powder. Roast in the oven for 20 minutes.

After 20 minutes, add the chickpeas and roast for another 15 minutes.

Remove from the oven and stir in the coconut milk, let sit for a few minutes for the flavours to meld together.

Nutritional values (Per serving, in g): Calories: 295, Fat: 10g, Sodium: 300mg, Carbs: 45g, Fiber: 12g, Protein: 9g

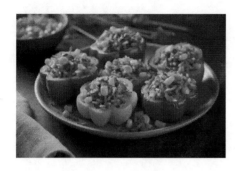

★ **Recipe 5: Vegan Stuffed Bell Peppers**

- Preparation Time: 45 minutes

- Serving: 4

- Method of Cooking: Baking

Ingredients:

- 4 bell peppers
- 1 cup cooked brown rice
- 1 zucchini (diced)
- 1 can low-sodium diced tomatoes
- 1 cup corn
- 1/2 cup low-sodium vegetable broth

Procedure:

Preheat the oven to 375°F (190°C). Cut off the tops of the peppers and remove the seeds.

In a large bowl, combine brown rice, chopped zucchini, diced tomatoes, and corn.

Stuff each bell pepper with the rice mixture. Place the peppers in a baking dish and pour the broth into the bottom of the dish.

Bake for 30-35 minutes until the peppers are tender.

Nutritional values (Per serving, in g): Calories: 210, Fat: 2g, Sodium: 200mg, Carbs: 45g, Fiber: 8g, Protein: 7g

Chapter 8: Dinner Delights: Gourmet Evening Meals

8.1. Luxurious Seafood Creations

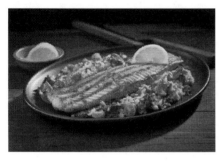

★ Recipe 1: Opulent Ocean Trout with Quinoa

- Preparation Time: 40 minutes

- Serving: 2

- Method of Cooking: Grilling and boiling

Ingredients:

- 2 Rainbow trout fillets
- 1 cup quinoa, rinsed
- 2 cups water
- Zest of 1 lemon
- 1 tbsp olive oil
- Salt to taste

Procedure:

Preheat grill to medium-high heat. Season rainbow trout fillets with a small pinch of salt and grill each side for 3-5 minutes.

Meanwhile, bring water to a boil in a pot. Add quinoa and reduce heat to low, let simmer for 15 minutes. Stir in olive oil and lemon zest.

Serve the grilled trout with a side of lemon-infused quinoa.

Nutritional values (estimated, in g): Calories: 460, Fat: 20g, Sodium: 190mg, Carbs: 40g, Fiber: 5g, Protein: 30g

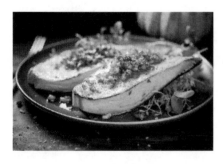

★ Recipe 2: Palace-Worthy Pollock over Roasted Acorn Squash

- Preparation Time: 45 minutes

- Serving: 2

- Method of Cooking: Baking

Ingredients:

- 2 Pollock fillets
- 1 small acorn squash, cut into quarters, seeds removed
- 1 tbsp olive oil
- A small pinch of Thyme
- Salt to taste

Procedure:

Preheat oven to 400°F (200°C). Place Pollock fillets and quarters of acorn squash on a baking sheet lined with parchment paper. Brush with olive oil and season with a small pinch of salt. Sprinkle acorn squash with thyme.

Bake for 25-30 minutes. Serve the baked Pollock over a wedge of roasted acorn squash.

Nutritional values (estimated, in g): Calories: 300, Fat: 10g, Sodium: 190mg, Carbs: 20g, Fiber: 3g, Protein: 35g

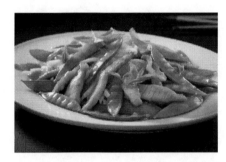

★ Recipe 3: Savory Sole Stir-fry with Snow Peas

- Preparation Time: 30 minutes

- Serving: 3

- Method of Cooking: Stir-frying

Ingredients:

- 2 Sole fillets, sliced into strips
- 1 cup snow peas
- 1 tbsp olive oil
- Salt to taste

Procedure:

Heat a wok or large frying pan over medium-high heat. Add olive oil and sole strips, stirring often until fish is cooked through, about 3-4 minutes. Remove fish and set aside. In the same pan, add snow peas and stir-fry for an additional 3-4 minutes until they are bright green but still crisp. Return fish to the pan, add a small pinch of salt, mix for about a minute, then serve.

Nutritional values (estimated, in g): Calories: 220, Fat: 10g, Sodium: 190mg, Carbs: 5g, Fiber: 2g, Protein: 30g

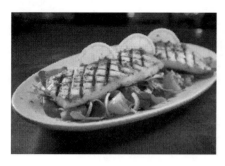

★ Recipe 4: Majestic Mahi Mahi over Mixed Greens

- Preparation Time: 30 minutes
- Serving: 2
- Method of Cooking: Grilling

Ingredients:

- 2 Mahi Mahi fillets
- 2 servings of mixed salad greens (about 4 cups)
- 2 tbsp vinaigrette, low sodium
- Salt to taste

Procedure:

Preheat grill to medium-high heat. Season Mahi Mahi fillets with a small pinch of salt and grill each side for 4-6 minutes.

Toss the mixed salad greens with the vinaigrette. Plate the salad and place the grilled Mahi Mahi atop the salad greens.

Nutritional values (estimated, in g): Calories: 240, Fat: 10g, Sodium: 200mg, Carbs: 5g, Fiber: 2g, Protein: 30g

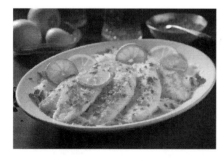

★ Recipe 5: Delicate Dory in Zesty Citrus Sauce

- Preparation Time: 20 minutes
- Serving: 2
- Method of Cooking: Pan-fryin

Ingredients:

- 2 Dory fillets
- Juice and zest of 1/2 lemon and 1/2 orange
- 1 tbsp olive oil
- Salt to taste

Procedure:

Preheat a skillet over medium-high heat. Brush Dory fillets with olive oil, season lightly with salt and pan-fry each side for 2-3 minutes.

Add the citrus juice to the pan, swirl around for another 2-3 minutes. Remove from the heat, sprinkle with zest and serve.

Nutritional values (estimated, in g): Calories: 300, Fat: 15g, Sodium: 250mg, Carbs: 5g, Fiber: 1g, Protein: 35g

8.2. Divine Meat Dishes

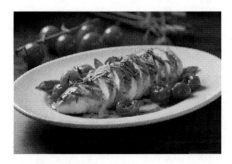

★ Recipe 1: Gourmet Stuffed Chicken with Roasted Cherry Tomatoes

- Preparation Time: 50 minutes

- Serving: 2

- Method of Cooking: Baking and roasting

Ingredients:

- 2 boneless skinless chicken breasts
- 1/2 cup low-sodium goat cheese
- 2 cups cherry tomatoes
- 2 tbsp olive oil
- Salt to taste

Procedure:

Preheat oven to 375°F (190°C). Cut a horizontal pocket into each chicken breast, making sure not to slice all the way through.

Stuff the chicken breast pockets with low-sodium goat cheese and secure the edges with toothpicks. Season exterior lightly with salt.

Arrange chicken breasts on a baking sheet alongside cherry tomatoes, drizzling olive oil over them.

Bake for 35-40 minutes, or until juices from the chicken run clear and the tomatoes are soft and bursting. Remove toothpicks before serving.

Nutritional values (estimated, in g): Calories: 430, Fat: 25g, Sodium: 280mg, Carbs: 20g, Fiber: 2g, Protein: 35g.

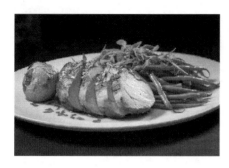

★ Recipe 2: Herb–Crusted Pork Tenderloin with Green Beans

- Preparation Time: 40 minutes

- Serving: 4

- Method of Cooking: Baking

Ingredients:

- 1 lb pork tenderloin
- 2 tbsp Dijon mustard, low-sodium
- 2 cups green beans, trimmed
- 1/2 cup mixed chopped herbs (rosemary, thyme, parsley)

- 2 tbsp olive oil
- Salt to taste

Procedure:

Preheat oven to 425°F (220°C). Rub the surface of pork tenderloin with a light layer of low-sodium Dijon mustard, sprinkle with mixed chopped herbs, and season lightly with salt.

Place the pork tenderloin on a baking sheet with a wire rack alongside green beans, drizzling olive oil over the beans.

Bake for 25-30 minutes or until internal temperature reaches 145-160°F (63-71°C).

Allow the tenderloin to rest for 10 minutes, then slice and serve with green beans.

Nutritional values (estimated, in g): Calories: 345, Fat: 15g, Sodium: 300mg, Carbs: 15g, Fiber: 4g, Protein: 40g.

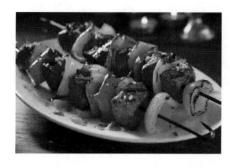

★ **Recipe 3: Mediterranean Beef Kabobs with Bell Peppers**

- Preparation Time: 25 minutes

- Serving: 4

- Method of Cooking: Grilling

Ingredients:

- 1 lb lean beef, cubed
- 2 Bell peppers (1 red, 1 yellow), cut into 1.5-inch squares
- 2 tbsp olive oil
- Salt to taste

Procedure:

Preheat grill to medium-high heat.

Skewer the cubed beef and bell pepper squares, alternating between them. Brush skewers with olive oil and season lightly with salt. Grill for 10-12 minutes, turning as needed to cook evenly. Serve the kabobs as they are or remove the meat and vegetables from the skewers. Nutritional values (estimated, in g): Calories: 380, Fat: 20g, Sodium: 250mg, Carbs: 10g, Fiber: 2g, Protein: 40g.

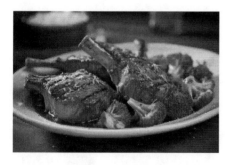

★ **Recipe 4: Garlic Rosemary Lamb Chops with Steamed Broccoli**

- Preparation Time: 30 minutes

- Serving: 2

- Method of Cooking: Pan-frying and steaming

Ingredients:

- 4 lamb chops
- 1 clove garlic, minced
- 1 tbsp chopped fresh rosemary
- 1 tbsp olive oil
- 2 cups broccoli florets
- Salt to taste

Procedure:

In a small bowl, mix olive oil, minced garlic, chopped rosemary, and a small pinch of salt. Marinate lamb chops in the mixture for 20 minutes.

Pan fry the marinated lamb chops over medium-high heat for 4-5 minutes per side, or until desired doneness is achieved.

Steam the broccoli florets in a steamer basket, covered, over simmering water for 5 minutes until tender.

Serve the lamb chops with a side of steamed broccoli.

Nutritional values (estimated, in g): Calories: 415, Fat: 25g, Sodium: 230mg, Carbs: 10g, Fiber: 4g, Protein: 40g.

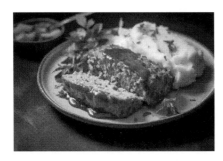

★ Recipe 5: Savory Turkey Roll-ups with Caramelized Onions

- Preparation Time: 60 minutes

- Serving: 4-6

- Method of Cooking: Baking and sautéing

Ingredients:

- 1 lb ground turkey
- 1 egg
- 1/2 cup breadcrumbs, low-sodium

- 2 large onions, thinly sliced
- 2 tbsp olive oil
- Salt to taste

Procedure:

Preheat oven to 350°F (175°C).

In a skillet, heat 1 tbsp of olive oil over medium-low heat. Cook sliced onions, stirring occasionally, for 25-30 minutes or until caramelized and golden brown. Set aside.

In a bowl, mix ground turkey, egg, breadcrumbs, caramelized onions, and a small pinch of salt, until evenly combined.

Shape the mixture into a loaf and transfer onto a parchment-lined baking sheet. Lightly brush with remaining olive oil. Bake for 40-45 minutes, or until internal temperature reaches 165°F (74°C). Remove from oven, let cool slightly, then slice and serve.

Nutritional values (estimated, in g): Calories: 380, Fat: 20g, Sodium: 250mg, Carbs: 20g, Fiber: 2g, Protein: 35g.

8.3. Elegant Vegetarian and Vegan Entrees

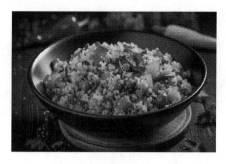

★ Recipe 1: Quinoa and Vegetable Stir-Fry

- Preparation Time: 30 minutes

- Serving: 4

- Method of Cooking: Stir-frying

Ingredients:

- 1 cup quinoa
- 2 cups water
- 1 tbsp olive oil
- 2 cloves garlic, minced
- 1 medium onion, sliced

- 1 bell pepper, julienned
- 3 stalks celery, diced
- 1/2 cup snow peas
- 2 tbsp low-sodium soy sauce
- Salt to taste

Procedure:Rinse the quinoa under cold water until water runs clear.

Bring 2 cups of water to a boil and add quinoa. Simmer for around 15 minutes, or until all water is absorbed. Set quinoa aside. In a wok, heat olive oil and sauté garlic and onions until translucent. Add bell pepper, celery, and snow peas, stirring frequently. After vegetables are tender, stir in the cooked quinoa and low sodium soy sauce. Cook for an additional 2-3 minutes, then remove from heat. Add salt to taste.

Nutritional values (estimated, in g): Calories: 285, Fat: 7g, Sodium: 240mg, Carbs: 48g, Fiber: 6g, Protein: 10g.

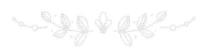

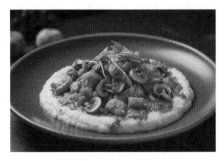

★ Recipe 2: Chickpea Mushroom Ragu with Polenta

- Preparation Time: 40 minutes

- Serving: 4

- Method of Cooking: Simmering and boiling

Ingredients:

- 1 cup polenta
- 4 cups water
- 1 can (400g) chickpeas, rinsed and drained
- 200g mushrooms, sliced
- 1 medium onion, diced

- 2 cloves garlic, minced
- 3 cups low-sodium vegetable broth
- Fresh parsley, chopped for garnishing
- Salt to taste

Procedure: Boil 4 cups of water in a pot, then gradually whisk in the polenta. Reduce heat to low and continue whisking until the polenta is thickened. In a skillet, sauté onion until translucent, then add the minced garlic and cook for another minute. Add mushrooms and cook until browned. Stir in chickpeas and low-sodium vegetable broth. Simmer for 15 minutes.

Pour the ragu over cooked polenta. Sprinkle with fresh parsley and add salt to taste.

Nutritional values (estimated, in g): Calories: 325, Fat: 5g, Sodium: 160mg, Carbs: 62g, Fiber: 10g, Protein: 12g.

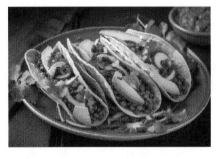

★ Recipe 3: Lentil Tacos with Avocado Salsa

- Preparation Time: 35 minutes

- Serving: 4 ((2 tacos each)

- Method of Cooking: Simmering

Ingredients:

- 1 cup lentils, rinsed
- 2 cups water

- 1 avocado, chopped
- 1 tomato, diced

- 1/2 red onion, diced
- 1/2 cup fresh cilantro, chopped
- Juice of one lime

- 2 bell peppers, sliced
- 8 taco shells
- Salt to taste

Procedure:

In a saucepan, bring water to a boil and add lentils. Cover and simmer until lentils are tender. Drain excess water.

In a bowl, combine avocado, tomato, red onion, cilantro, and lime juice to make the avocado salsa. Add salt to season.

Assemble tacos by spooning lentils and avocado salsa into each taco shell.

Serve with a side of bell pepper slices.

Nutritional values (estimated, in g): Calories: 410, Fat: 12g, Sodium: 120mg, Carbs: 67g, Fiber: 23g, Protein: 20g.

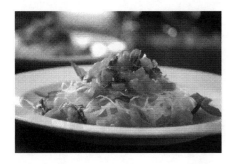

★ Recipe 4: Spaghetti Squash with Tomato Basil Sauce

- Preparation Time: 50 minutes
- Serving: 4
- Method of Cooking: Baking

Ingredients:

- 1 spaghetti squash, cut in half lengthwise
- 1 can (400g) no-salt-added diced tomatoes
- 2 cloves garlic, minced

- 1 onion, diced
- 1/4 cup fresh basil, chopped
- 1 tsp olive oil
- Salt to taste

Procedure: Preheat oven to 375°F (190°C). Place spaghetti squash halves, cut-side down, on a baking sheet. Bake until tender, about 40 minutes. Heat olive oil in a pan on medium heat. Sauté onions and garlic until translucent. Add diced tomatoes and simmer for about 10 minutes. Stir in chopped basil. Once spaghetti squash is cooked, use a fork to shred the inside, creating "spaghetti". Serve with tomato-basil sauce and salt.

Nutritional values (estimated, in g): Calories: 175, Fat: 3.5g, Sodium: 45mg, Carbs: 39g, Fiber: 2g, Protein: 3g.

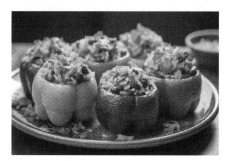

★ **Recipe 5: Bean and Rice Stuffed Bell Peppers**

- Preparation Time: 60 minutes

- Serving: 4

- Method of Cooking: Baking and Boiling

Ingredients:

- 4 bell peppers, tops removed and seeded
- 1 cup brown rice
- 2 cups water
- 1 cup black beans, rinsed and drained

- 1 onion, diced
- 2 cloves garlic, minced
- 1 tsp ground cumin
- Salt to taste

Procedure: Preheat oven to 375°F (190°C).

In a saucepan, bring 2 cups of water to a boil and add rice. Simmer until rice is cooked. Mix cooked rice with black beans, onion, garlic, and cumin. Stuff each bell pepper with the rice and bean mixture. Place stuffed peppers in a baking dish and bake for about 25 minutes. Serve with a pinch of salt.

Nutritional values (estimated, in g): Calories: 345, Fat: 3g, Sodium: 10mg, Carbs: 72g, Fiber: 14g, Protein: 12g.

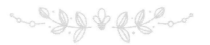

Chapter 9: Snacks and Munchies: Savor the In-between Moments

9.1. Nutritious Dips and Spreads

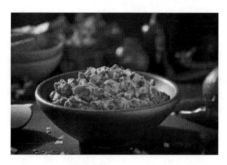

★ Recipe 1: Creamy Avocado Dip

- Preparation Time: 10 minutes

- Serving: 4

- Method of Cooking: Blending

Ingredients:

- 2 ripe avocados
- 1 small clove garlic, minced
- 1 tbsp fresh lime juice
- Salt to taste

Procedure:Halve avocados, remove the pits, and scoop out the flesh. In a blender, combine avocado, garlic, and lime juice. Blend until completely smooth. Season with salt to taste. Nutritional values (estimated, in g): Calories: 120, Fat: 10g, Sodium: 5mg, Carbs: 8g, Fiber: 6g, Protein: 2g.

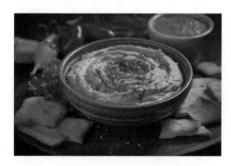

★ Recipe 2: Roasted Red Pepper Hummus

- Preparation Time: 15 minutes

- Serving: 8

- Method of Cooking: Blending

Ingredients:

- 1 can (400g) low sodium chickpeas, drained and rinsed
- 2 roasted red peppers
- 2 cloves garlic, minced
- 2 tbsp olive oil
- 2 tbsp fresh lemon juice
- Salt to taste

Procedure: In a blender or food processor, combine chickpeas, roasted red peppers, garlic, olive oil, and lemon juice. Blend until smooth. Season with salt to taste. Nutritional values (estimated, in g): Calories: 80, Fat: 4g, Sodium: 30mg, Carbs: 10g, Fiber: 3g, Protein: 3g.

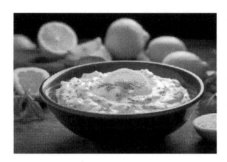

★ Recipe 3: Tangy Greek Yogurt Dip

- Preparation Time: 5 minutes

- Serving: 8

- Method of Cooking: Mixing

Ingredients:

- 2 cups unsalted Greek yogurt
- 1 clove garlic, minced
- 1 tsp fresh dill, chopped

- 1 tbsp fresh lemon juice
- Salt to taste

Procedure: In a mixing bowl, combine Greek yogurt, garlic, dill, and lemon juice. Stir until fully blended, season with salt to taste. Allow flavors to meld in refrigerator for at least one hour before serving. Nutritional values (estimated, in g): Calories: 45, Fat: 1g, Sodium: 15mg, Carbs: 2g, Fiber: 0g, Protein: 7g.

9.2. Crunchy and Satisfying Treats

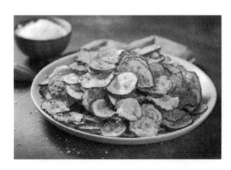

★ Recipe 1: Baked Zucchini Chips

- Preparation Time: 35 minutes

- Serving: 4

- Method of Cooking: Baking

Ingredients:

- 2 zucchinis, sliced into thin rounds
- 1 tbsp olive oil

- 1/2 tsp dried oregano
- Salt to tast

Procedure:

Preheat the oven to 225°F (105°C) and line a baking sheet with parchment paper. Toss the zucchini slices with olive oil, dried oregano, and a pinch of salt. Arrange the slices on the baking sheet in a single layer. Bake for 2 hours or until crisp and golden. Cool before serving. Nutritional values (estimated, in g): Calories: 60, Fat: 3.5g, Sodium: 5mg, Carbs: 6g, Fiber: 2g, Protein: 2g.

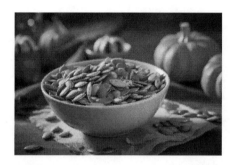

★ Recipe 2: Toasted Pumpkin Seeds

- Preparation Time: 45 minutes

- Serving: 8

- Method of Cooking: Toasting

Ingredients:

- 1 cup raw pumpkin seeds, rinsed and dried
- 1 tbsp olive oil
- Salt to taste
- Servings: 4

Procedure: Preheat the oven to 300°F (150°C) and line a baking sheet with parchment paper. Toss the pumpkin seeds with the olive oil and a pinch of salt. Spread the seeds out on the baking sheet in a single layer. Toast in the oven for about 40-45 minutes or until golden brown, stirring occasionally. Nutritional values (estimated, in g): Calories: 180, Fat: 15g, Sodium: 5mg, Carbs: 4g, Fiber: 2g, Protein: 9g.

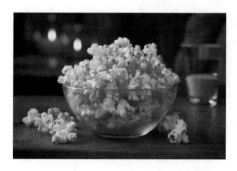

★ Recipe 3: Honey Cinnamon Popcorn

- Preparation Time: 5 minutes

- Serving: 4

- Method of Cooking: Mix, Heat

Ingredients:

- 4 cups air-popped popcorn
- 1 tbsp honey

- 1/2 tsp ground cinnamon

Procedure:

Heat the honey until it becomes runny. Toss the popcorn with the heated honey and ground cinnamon until coated evenly. Allow it to cool before serving.

Nutritional values (estimated, in g): Calories: 70, Fat: 1g, Sodium: 0mg, Carbs: 15g, Fiber: 3g, Protein: 2g.

9.3. Fruit and Vegetable Snacks

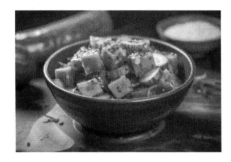

★ Recipe 1: Refreshing Watermelon Salad

- Preparation Time: 10 minutes

- Serving: 4

- Method of Cooking: Raw/Toss

Ingredients:

- 2 cups watermelon cubes
- 1 cup cucumber slices
- 1 tbsp fresh mint, chopped
- Juice of 1 lime

Procedure: In a large bowl, combine watermelon cubes and cucumber slices. Sprinkle chopped mint over the watermelon and cucumber. Drizzle lime juice over the top. Chill in the refrigerator before serving. Nutritional values (estimated, in g): Calories: 35, Fat: 0g, Sodium: 0mg, Carbs: 8g, Fiber: 1g, Protein: 1g.

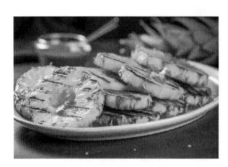

★ Recipe 2: Grilled Pineapple Spears

- Preparation Time: 15 minutes

- Serving: 4

- Method of Cooking: Grilling

Ingredients:

- 1 ripe pineapple, cut into spears
- 1 tbsp honey
- Juice of 1 lime

Procedure: Preheat the grill to medium-high. In a small bowl, combine honey and lime juice. Brush the pineapple spears with the honey and lime mixture. Grill for around 10 minutes, turning occasionally, until caramelized and slightly charred.

Nutritional values (estimated, in g): Calories: 80, Fat: 0g, Sodium: 0mg, Carbs: 21g, Fiber: 2g, Protein: 1g.

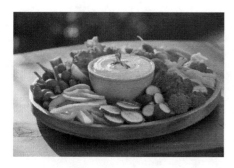

★ Recipe 3: Crunchy Veggie Sticks with Herb Yogurt Dip

- Preparation Time: 10 minutes

- Serving: 4

- Method of Cooking: Raw/Mixing

Ingredients:

- 2 cups mixed raw vegetables (cucumber, bell peppers), cut into sticks
- 1 cup unsalted Greek yogurt
- 2 tbsp fresh herbs (parsley, dill), chopped
- 1 clove garlic, minced
- Juice of 1 lemon

Procedure: Arrange vegetables on a plate. In a bowl, combine Greek yogurt, herbs, garlic, and lemon juice. Chill the dip in the refrigerator before serving with the raw vegetables. Nutritional values (estimated, in g): Calories: 70, Fat: 1g, Sodium: 30mg, Carbs: 7g, Fiber: 2g, Protein: 9g.

Chapter 10: Dessert Delights: Sweet Treats for a Kidney-Friendly Diet

10.1. Easy No-Bake Desserts

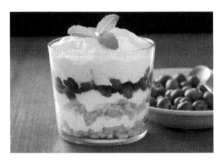

★ Recipe 1: Luscious Lemon Blueberry Parfait

- Preparation Time: 15 minutes

- Serving: 4

- Method of Cooking: Layering/Mixing

Ingredients:

- 2 cups low-fat vanilla Greek yogurt
- 1 cup fresh blueberries
- Zest and juice of 1 lemon
- 1 tbsp honey

Procedure: In a bowl, mix together Greek yogurt, lemon zest, and honey. In 4 serving glasses, alternate layers of the yogurt mixture and fresh blueberries. Chill in the refrigerator for at least 1 hour before serving. Nutritional values (estimated, in g): Calories: 110, Fat: 1g, Sodium: 40mg, Carbs: 15g, Fiber: 1g, Protein: 10g.

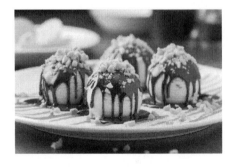

★ Recipe 2: Creamy Peanut Butter Banana Bites

- Preparation Time: 20 minutes (plus freezing)

- Serving: 4 (8-10 bites)

- Method of Cooking: Freezing

Ingredients:

- 2 ripe bananas
- 4 tbsp peanut butter, unsalted
- 2 tbsp honey
- Dark chocolate shavings for topping

Procedure:

Slice the bananas into half-inch slices. Spread a thin layer of peanut butter on half the slices, drizzle with honey and cover with other banana slice. Place the bites onto a lined baking sheet or a plate and freeze for at least 2 hours or until firm. Serve with a sprinkle of dark chocolate shavings on top.

Nutritional values (estimated, in g): Calories: 140, Fat: 6g, Sodium: 30mg, Carbs: 20g, Fiber: 3g, Protein: 3g.

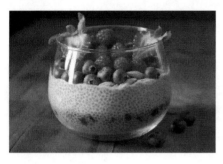

★ Recipe 3: Chia Berry Pudding

- Preparation Time: 10 minutes (plus chilling)

- Serving: 4

- Method of Cooking: Mixing/Refrigeration

Ingredients:

- 2 cups almond milk, unsweetened
- 1/2 cup chia seeds
- 1 cup mixed berries
- 2 tbsp honey

Procedure:In a large bowl, whisk together almond milk and chia seeds. Let sit for 5 minutes, then whisk again. Refrigerate the mixture for at least 1 hour or overnight until it becomes a gel-like pudding. When ready to serve, sweeten with honey and top with mixed berries.Nutritional values (estimated, in g): Calories: 200, Fat: 9g, Sodium: 90mg, Carbs: 24g, Fiber: 12g, Protein: 7g.

10.2. Healthier Takes on Classic Desserts

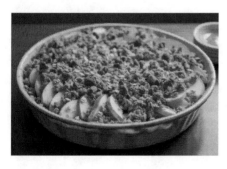

★ Recipe 1: Apple Crumble Delight

- Preparation Time: 20 minutes

- Serving: 4

- Method of Cooking: Baking

Ingredients:

- 4 cups apples, peeled, cored, and sliced thinly
- 1/2 cup rolled oats
- 3 tbsp almond flour
- 2 tbsp unsalted butter, chilled and cubed

- 1/4 cup honey
- 1/4 tsp cinnamon

Procedure:

Preheat oven to 350°F (180°C).

In a medium-sized mixing bowl, combine rolled oats, almond flour, cinnamon, and chilled butter. Mix until the mixture resembles coarse crumbs. Arrange apple slices in a lightly greased 8x8-inch baking dish. Drizzle honey on top of the sliced apples. Sprinkle the crumble mixture evenly across the top of the apples. Bake for 30-35 minutes or until the apples are tender and the topping is golden brown.

Nutritional values (estimated, in g): Calories: 270, Fat: 9g, Sodium: 5mg, Carbs: 47g, Fiber: 5g, Protein: 3g.

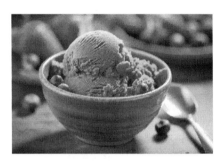

★ **Recipe 2: Zesty Berry Sorbet**

- Preparation Time: 15 minutes (plus freezing)
- Serving: 4
- Method of Cooking: Blending/Freezing

Ingredients:

- 4 cups mixed berries (raspberries, strawberries, and blueberries), frozen
- 1/2 cup honey
- 1/2 cup water
- Zest and juice from 1 lemon

Procedure:

In a blender or food processor, combine the frozen mixed berries, honey, water, lemon zest, and lemon juice. Blend until smooth. Pour into a loaf tin or airtight container, and freeze for at least 4 hours, or overnight. Scoop and serve!

Nutritional values (estimated, in g): Calories: 180, Fat: 1g, Sodium: 5mg, Carbs: 44g, Fiber: 5g, Protein: 1g.

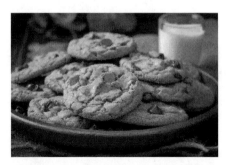

★ **Recipe 3: Whole Wheat Chocolate Chip Cookies**

- Preparation Time: 15 minutes
- Serving: 18 cookies

- Method of Cooking: Mixing/Freezing

Ingredients:

- 1 cup whole-wheat flour
- 1/4 tsp baking soda
- 1/8 tsp salt
- 1/4 cup unsalted butter, room temperature
- 1/4 cup honey
- 1 egg
- 1/2 cup dark chocolate chips

Procedure:

Preheat oven to 350°F (180°C). Line a baking sheet with parchment paper.

In a bowl, whisk together whole wheat flour, baking soda, and salt.

In another bowl, beat butter and honey until creamy.

Beat the egg into the butter mixture.

Gradually add the dry ingredients into the wet ingredients, mixing until combined.

Fold in the chocolate chips.

Drop heaping tablespoons of cookie dough onto the prepared baking sheet.

Bake for 10-12 minutes or until the edges are lightly golden.

Allow to cool on the baking sheet for a few minutes before transferring to a wire rack to cool completely.

Nutritional values (estimated, in g): Calories: 92, Fat: 4g, Sodium: 35mg, Carbs: 13g, Fiber: 1g, Protein: 1g.

Chapter 11: Beverages and Alcohol: Quenching Thirst the Right Way

11.1. Kidney-Friendly Hydration

It's time to comprehend the significance of beverages and alcohol in a kidney-friendly diet. Keeping hydrated is vital for maintaining overall health, but it's equally essential to choose the right type of drinks that aid kidney function without causing harm.

Understanding Kidney-Friendly Drinks

Stay away from excessive amounts of sugar, sodium, and phosphorus, even when seeking hydration. Patients with kidney disease, especially in advanced stages, need to keep fluid intake in check as the kidneys may struggle to regulate fluid balance.

Water: The Best Choice for Hydration

Water remains the most crucial source of hydration for everybody, including individuals with kidney problems. It helps regulate body temperature, flush waste products, support digestion and absorption, and maintain fluid balance. Patients with kidney disease should consult their healthcare providers for personalized advice on the daily intake of water, as the recommended quantity may vary depending on the stage of the disease.

Why Herbal Teas Make a Difference

Herbal teas, specifically those low in potassium and phosphorus, can be a fitting addition to the diet. Incorporating teas like chamomile, lemon, hibiscus, and mint can gradually improve overall health. These teas possess anti-inflammatory and antioxidant properties, rendering them beneficial for kidney function. When preparing your herbal tea, be sure to avoid using teas with a high mineral content, such as dandelion or nettle tea, and forgo sugar or honey to maintain their low calorie count.

Fruit Infused Waters: Creative and Healthy Concoctions

By combining hydration and nourishment, you can simultaneously indulge the taste buds and take care of your renal health. For a delightful and refreshing fruit infusion, try using low-potassium fruits such as apples, raspberries, blueberries, or pineapple with purified water. Additionally, you may experiment with different combinations to find the taste that suits your palate.

The Wholesome Goodness of Nut Milk and Rice Milk

For a kidney-conscious diet, opting for nut milk and rice milk can be a wise decision. These dairy alternatives excel as nutrient-dense drinks devoid of phosphorus and potassium. You can prepare homemade almond or cashew milk by blending soaked nuts with fresh water in a high-powered blender, then straining the mixture to extract the milk. However, exercise caution when purchasing store-bought nut milk, as some may contain added salt and phosphorus.

The Role of Low-Sodium & Homemade Vegetable Juices

Though fruit juices typically contain high sugar and potassium levels, vegetable juices offer a valuable alternative by providing low-sodium, homemade options. Freshly-prepared and low-sodium vegetable juices can help maintain kidney health by offering essential vitamins and minerals, without an overload of sodium or potassium. Consider juicing a mix of vegetables, such as cucumber, zucchini, bell pepper, and leafy greens. Adding a slice of lemon or a dash of recommended herbs and spices can give your juice an extra burst of flavor.

11.2. Healthy and Tasty Alternatives to Sugary Drinks

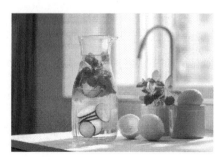

★ Recipe 1: Refreshing Cucumber–Mint Cooler

- Preparation Time: 15 minutes

- Serving: 2

Ingredients:

- One whole cucumber (sliced)
- A handful of fresh mint leaves
- Juice of half a lemon
- Two cups of water
- Ice cubes for serving

Procedure:

In a blender, combine the sliced cucumber, fresh mint leaves, and lemon juice. Blend until smooth.

Pour the mixture through a fine-mesh sieve into a jug filled with water, pressing down on the solids to extract as much juice as possible. Discard the solids.

Stir the mixture well and refrigerate for an hour before serving.

Serve chilled in glasses filled with ice cubes.

Nutritional values: (per serving) Calories: 15, Protein: 0.5g, Fat: 0g , Carbohydrates:3.5g, Sodium: 2mg, Potassium: 75mg

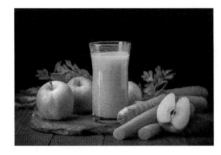

★ **Recipe 2: Invigorating Carrot-Apple-Ginger Juice**
- Preparation Time: 10 minutes
- Serving: 2

Ingredients:

- Two apples, cored
- Four carrots, peeled
- One inch of fresh ginger root

Procedure:

Thoroughly wash the cored apples, peeled carrots, and ginger root.

Using a juicer, extract the juice from the apples, carrots, and ginger.

Stir the freshly pressed juice and divide between two glasses. Serve immediately.

Nutritional values: (per serving) Calories: 95, Protein: 0.5g, Fat: 0.3g, Carbohydrates: 23g, Sodium: 40mg, Potassium: 55mg

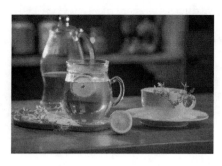

★ Recipe 3: Soothing Chamomile-Lemon Hot Tea

- Preparation Time: 10 minutes

- Serving: 2

Ingredients:

- Two cups of water
- Two bags of chamomile tea
- Half a lemon (juiced)

Procedure:

In a saucepan, bring the water to a boil.

Once boiling, remove from the heat and steep the chamomile tea bags in the hot water for five minutes.

Squeeze in the juice of half a lemon. Stir to combine.

Pour the hot tea into two mugs, and serve immediately.

Nutritional values: (per serving) Calories: 2, Protein: 0g, Fat: 0g, Carbohydrates: 0.5g, Sodium: 0mg, Potassium: 5mg

11.3. Alcohol Use in the Renal Diet

Alcohol, in moderation, has been often viewed as a socially acceptable beverage choice. Whether it's a glass of wine accompanying dinner or a pint of beer shared with friends, alcoholic beverages tend to form an integral part of our social gatherings. But when it comes to kidney health, can alcohol fit safely into a renal diet?

While moderate alcohol consumption doesn't cause kidney disease per se, excessive indulgence certainly creates risk factors inclining one towards renal issues. High blood pressure, liver disease, and improper hydration, induced by overconsumption, can lead to a cascading chain of events, contributing to declining kidney health.

Moderation is Key: Renal Diet and Alcohol

When we talk about a renal diet, the primary goal is to manage the consumption of proteins, sodium, potassium, phosphorus, and fluids. Alcohol doesn't significantly impact these quintessential facets directly, but its influence on overall health can alter their management.

Thus, integrating alcohol into a renal diet is very much a question of keeping its consumption moderate and well within the boundaries of your health status. People with kidney disease should limit alcohol use to occasional, moderate drinking, or avoid it altogether, depending on their specific health circumstances.

The Typology of Alcoholic Beverages

The type of beverage chosen also plays a role in the relationship between alcoholic beverages and kidney health. Not all drinks are created equal. Beers and some types of liquor can be high in phosphorus, something those with kidney issues need to limit.

On the other hand, while some wines may be lower in phosphorus, they can be high in potassium, another mineral that can be harmful to those with kidney disease if consumed in excess. Furthermore, cocktails and mixed drinks can contain high amounts of sodium and sugar, both of which can negatively affect a renal diet.

Enhancing Mindfulness: Your Role in Monitoring

Apart from open communication with your health professional, it's crucial to foster etiquettes of mindful drinking. You need to be aware of the potency of your drinks, serving sizes, and keep track of the number of drinks you're having. Essentially, alcohol should not be seen as a thirst quencher; it's an added beverage that demands consciousness while consuming.

Living with kidney disease and adapting to a renal diet doesn't mean you have to miss out on the joys of life. It's about making mindful, measured choices to enhance your health without compromising much on enjoyment.

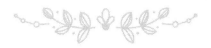

Chapter 12: 90-Day Meal Schedule

12.1:Beginning of the Journey: The First Month

WEEK 1	Monday	Tuesday	Wednesday	Thursday	Friday	Saturday	Sunday
Breakfast	Morning Zest Smoothie	Sunny Quinoa Bowl	Tofu Scramble	Blueberry Avocado Delight	Banana Nut Overnight Oats	Vegan Quinoa Porridge	Cinnamon Apple Oats Smoothie
Lunch	Spicy Avocado and Chickpea Sandwich	Tangy Citrus and Fennel Salad	Chicken and Wild Rice Soup	Veggie Hummus Wrap	Grilled Asparagus and Chickpea Salad	Kidney-Friendly BLT	Creamy Butternut Squash Soup
Snack	Grilled Pineapple Spears	Apple Crumble Delight	Creamy Avocado Dip	Whole Wheat Chocolate Chip Cookies	Refreshing Watermelon Salad	Chia Berry Pudding	Toasted Pumpkin Seeds
Dinner	Opulent Ocean Trout with Quinoa	Spaghetti Squash with Tomato Basil Sauce	Quinoa and Vegetable Stir-Fry	Savory Sole Stir-fry with Snow Peas	Herb-Crusted Pork Tenderloin with Green Beans	Chickpea Mushroom Ragu with Polenta	Palace-Worthy Pollock over Roasted Acorn Squash

WEEK 2	Monday	Tuesday	Wednesday	Thursday	Friday	Saturday	Sunday
Breakfast	Veggie Egg White Scramble	Tropical Chia Pudding	Buckwheat Pancakes	Nourishing Nutty Delight	Low-Sodium Rice Cake with Avocado	Chia Berry Smoothie Bowl	Green Detox Smoothie
Lunch	Mediterranean Veggie Pita	Cucumber, Tomato, and Avocado Salad	Lentil and Vegetable Soup	Tofu Salad Sandwich	Greek Quinoa Salad	Spicy Avocado and Chickpea Sandwich	Chicken Noodle Soup
Snack	Luscious Lemon Blueberry Parfait	Apple Crumble Delight	Creamy Peanut Butter Banana Bites	Whole Wheat Chocolate Chip Cookies	Zesty Berry Sorbet	Chia Berry Pudding	Grilled Pineapple Spears
Dinner	Majestic Mahi Mahi over Mixed Greens	Mediterranean Beef Kabobs with Bell Peppers	Lentil Tacos with Avocado Salsa	Delicate Dory in Zesty Citrus Sauce	Garlic Rosemary Lamb Chops with Steamed Broccoli	Bean and Rice Stuffed Bell Peppers	Savory Turkey Roll-ups with Caramelized Onions

WEEK 3	Monday	Tuesday	Wednesday	Thursday	Friday	Saturday	Sunday
Breakfast	Blueberry Avocado Delight	Cinnamon Apple Oats Smoothie	Tofu Scramble	Green Detox Smoothie	Nourishing Nutty Delight	Morning Zest Smoothie	Cinnamon Apple Oats Smoothie
Lunch	Grilled Shrimp with Rosemary Lemon Sauce	Mediterranean Veggie Pita	Tuna Nicoise Salad	Chicken Noodle Soup	Lentil and Vegetable Soup	Grilled Shrimp with Rosemary Lemon Sauce	Mediterranean Veggie Pita
Snack	Creamy Avocado Dip with veggies	Baked Zucchini Chips	Tangy Greek Yogurt Dip with veggies	Easy Crab Cakes	Honey Cinnamon Popcorn	Refreshing Watermelon Salad	Quinoa Stuffed Bell Peppers
Dinner	Chicken Marsala with Sautéed Mushrooms	Quinoa and Lentil Salad	Spaghetti Squash with Tomato Basil Sauce	Grilled Lemon-Thyme Lamb Chops	Pan-Seared Cod with Sautéed Spinach	Quinoa Stuffed Bell Peppers	Veggie Tofu Stir-fry

WEEK 4	Monday	Tuesday	Wednesday	Thursday	Friday	Saturday	Sunday
Breakfast	Blueberry Avocado Delight	Tofu Scramble	Green Detox Smoothie	Nourishing Nutty Delight	Morning Zest Smoothie	Cinnamon Apple Oats Smoothie	Blueberry Avocado Delight
Lunch	Tuna Nicoise Salad	Chicken Noodle Soup	Lentil and Vegetable Soup	Grilled Shrimp with Rosemary Lemon Sauce	Mediterranean Veggie Pita	Tuna Nicoise Salad	Chicken Noodle Soup
Snack	Honey Cinnamon Popcorn	Roasted Red Pepper Hummus with veggies	Tangy Greek Yogurt Dip with veggies	Creamy Avocado Dip with veggies	Roasted Red Pepper Hummus with veggies	Toasted Pumpkin Seeds	Creamy Avocado Dip
Dinner	Herb-Crusted Pork Tenderloin with Green Beans	Quinoa and Vegetable Stir-Fry	Italian-Style Beef Ragu	Quinoa Stuffed Bell Peppers	Veggie Tofu Stir-fry	Grilled Lemon-Thyme Lamb Chops	Pan-Seared Cod with Sautéed Spinach

12.2: Continuing the Adventure: The Second Month

WEEK 1	Monday	Tuesday	Wednesday	Thursday	Friday	Saturday	Sunday
Breakfast	Tofu Scramble	Green Detox Smoothie	Nourishing Nutty Delight	Morning Zest Smoothie	Cinnamon Apple Oats Smoothie	Blueberry Avocado Delight	Sunny Quinoa Bowl
Lunch	Caramelized Onion and Mushroom Tart	Grilled Shrimp with Rosemary Lemon Sauce	Mediterranean Veggie Pita	Tuna Nicoise Salad	Chicken Noodle Soup	Easy Crab Cakes	Red Lentil and Sweet Potato Soup
Snack	Crunchy Veggie Sticks with Herb Yogurt Dip	Creamy Avocado Dip	Roasted Red Pepper Hummus with veggies	Tangy Greek Yogurt Dip with veggies	Honey Cinnamon Popcorn	Tangy Greek Yogurt Dip with veggies	Creamy Avocado Dip with veggies
Dinner	Lentil Tacos with Avocado Salsa	Savory Turkey Roll-ups with Caramelized Onions	Veggie Tofu Stir-fry	Grilled Lemon-Thyme Lamb Chops	Pan-Seared Cod with Sautéed Spinach	Italian-Style Beef Ragu	Quinoa Stuffed Bell Peppers

WEEK 2	Monday	Tuesday	Wednesday	Thursday	Friday	Saturday	Sunday
Breakfast	Green Detox Smoothie	Sunny Quinoa Bowl	Morning Zest Smoothie	Cinnamon Apple Oats Smoothie	Blueberry Avocado Delight	Green Detox Smoothie	Nourishing Nutty Delight
Lunch	Mediterranean Veggie Pita	Tuna Nicoise Salad	Chicken Noodle Soup	Lentil and Vegetable Soup	Grilled Shrimp with Rosemary Lemon Sauce	Quinoa Stuffed Bell Peppers	Cauliflower Fried "Rice"
Snack	Grilled Pineapple Spears	Tangy Greek Yogurt Dip with veggies	Roasted Red Pepper Hummus with veggies	Tangy Greek Yogurt Dip with veggies	Creamy Avocado Dip with veggies	Toasted Pumpkin Seeds	Baked Zucchini Chips
Dinner	Veggie Tofu Stir-fry	Grilled Lemon-Thyme Lamb Chops	Herb-Crusted Pork Tenderloin with Green Beans	Italian-Style Beef Ragu	Quinoa Stuffed Bell Peppers	Lentil Tacos with Avocado Salsa	Bean and Rice Stuffed Bell Peppers

WEEK 3	Monday	Tuesday	Wednesday	Thursday	Friday	Saturday	Sunday
Breakfast	Blueberry Avocado Delight	Cinnamon Apple Oats Smoothie	Tofu Scramble	Green Detox Smoothie	Nourishing Nutty Delight	Morning Zest Smoothie	Cinnamon Apple Oats Smoothie
Lunch	Grilled Shrimp with Rosemary Lemon Sauce	Mediterranean Veggie Pita	Tuna Nicoise Salad	Chicken Noodle Soup	Lentil and Vegetable Soup	Grilled Shrimp with Rosemary Lemon Sauce	Mediterranean Veggie Pita
Snack	Creamy Avocado Dip with veggies	Baked Zucchini Chips	Tangy Greek Yogurt Dip with veggies	Easy Crab Cakes	Honey Cinnamon Popcorn	Refreshing Watermelon Salad	Quinoa Stuffed Bell Peppers
Dinner	Chicken Marsala with Sautéed Mushrooms	Quinoa and Lentil Salad	Spaghetti Squash with Tomato Basil Sauce	Grilled Lemon-Thyme Lamb Chops	Pan-Seared Cod with Sautéed Spinach	Quinoa Stuffed Bell Peppers	Veggie Tofu Stir-fry

WEEK 4	Monday	Tuesday	Wednesday	Thursday	Friday	Saturday	Sunday
Breakfast	Blueberry Avocado Delight	Tofu Scramble	Green Detox Smoothie	Nourishing Nutty Delight	Morning Zest Smoothie	Cinnamon Apple Oats Smoothie	Blueberry Avocado Delight
Lunch	Tuna Nicoise Salad	Chicken Noodle Soup	Lentil and Vegetable Soup	Grilled Shrimp with Rosemary Lemon Sauce	Mediterranean Veggie Pita	Tuna Nicoise Salad	Chicken Noodle Soup
Snack	Honey Cinnamon Popcorn	Roasted Red Pepper Hummus with veggies	Tangy Greek Yogurt Dip with veggies	Creamy Avocado Dip with veggies	Roasted Red Pepper Hummus with veggies	Toasted Pumpkin Seeds	Creamy Avocado Dip
Dinner	Herb-Crusted Pork Tenderloin with Green Beans	Quinoa and Vegetable Stir-Fry	Italian-Style Beef Ragu	Quinoa Stuffed Bell Peppers	Veggie Tofu Stir-fry	Grilled Lemon-Thyme Lamb Chops	Pan-Seared Cod with Sautéed Spinach

12.3: The Final Stretch: The Third Month

WEEK 1	Monday	Tuesday	Wednesday	Thursday	Friday	Saturday	Sunday
Breakfast	Low-Sodium Rice Cake with Avocado	Morning Zest Smoothie	Tofu Scramble	Cinnamon Apple Oats Smoothie	Vegan Quinoa Porridge	Blueberry Avocado Delight	Buckwheat Pancakes
Lunch	Eggplant and Chickpea Stew	Grilled Asparagus and Chickpea Salad	Tuna Nicoise Salad	Vegetable Paella with Saffron	Cucumber, Tomato, and Avocado Salad	Poached Salmon with Asparagus	Cauliflower Fried "Rice"
Snack	Roasted Red Pepper Hummus	Toasted Pumpkin Seeds	Grilled Pineapple Spears	Tangy Greek Yogurt Dip	Honey Cinnamon Popcorn	Crunchy Veggie Sticks with Herb Yogurt Dip	Creamy Avocado Dip
Dinner	Delicate Dory in Zesty Citrus Sauce	Lentil Tacos with Avocado Salsa	Majestic Mahi Mahi over Mixed Greens	Gourmet Stuffed Chicken with Roasted Cherry Tomatoes	Spaghetti Squash with Tomato Basil Sauce	Delicate Dory in Zesty Citrus Sauce	Herb-Crusted Pork Tenderloin with Green Beans

WEEK 2	Monday	Tuesday	Wednesday	Thursday	Friday	Saturday	Sunday
Breakfast	Nourishing Nutty Delight	Chia Berry Smoothie Bowl	Green Detox Smoothie	Vegan Chickpea Omelette	Sunny Quinoa Bowl	Banana Nut Overnight Oats	Veggie Egg White Scramble
Lunch	Easy Crab Cakes	Caramelized Onion and Mushroom Tart	Tofu Salad Sandwich	Grilled Shrimp with Rosemary Lemon Sauce	Quinoa Stuffed Bell Peppers	Tangy Citrus and Fennel Salad	Pan-Seared Cod with Sautéed Spinach
Snack	Grilled Pineapple Spears	Tangy Greek Yogurt Dip	Honey Cinnamon Popcorn	Crunchy Veggie Sticks with Herb Yogurt Dip	Creamy Avocado Dip	Baked Zucchini Chips	Refreshing Watermelon Salad
Dinner	Opulent Ocean Trout with Quinoa	Savory Sole Stir-fry with Snow Peas	Quinoa and Vegetable Stir-Fry	Palace-Worthy Pollock over Roasted Acorn Squash	Majestic Mahi Mahi over Mixed Greens	Chickpea Mushroom Ragu with Polenta	Savory Sole Stir-fry with Snow Peas

WEEK 3	Monday	Tuesday	Wednesday	Thursday	Friday	Saturday	Sunday
Breakfast	Tropical Chia Pudding	Low-Sodium Rice Cake with Avocado	Morning Zest Smoothie	Tofu Scramble	Cinnamon Apple Oats Smoothie	Vegan Quinoa Porridge	Banana Nut Overnight Oats
Lunch	Veggie Hummus Wrap	Tuna Nicoise Salad	Vegetable Paella with Saffron	Kidney-Friendly BLT	Poached Salmon with Asparagus	Cauliflower Fried "Rice"	Mediterranean Veggie Pita
Snack	Honey Cinnamon Popcorn	Crunchy Veggie Sticks with Herb Yogurt Dip	Creamy Avocado Dip	Baked Zucchini Chips	Refreshing Watermelon Salad	Roasted Red Pepper Hummus	Toasted Pumpkin Seeds
Dinner	Garlic Butter Shrimp Skewers	Baked Sweet Potato and Black Bean Tacos	Roasted Pork Tenderloin with Rosemary and Garlic	Baked Salmon with Spinach Pesto	Roasted Cauliflower and Chickpea Curry	Tangy Balsamic Steak Stir-Fry	Sweet Chili Lime Grilled Shrimp

WEEK 4	Monday	Tuesday	Wednesday	Thursday	Friday	Saturday	Sunday
Breakfast	Blueberry Avocado Delight	Buckwheat Pancakes	Nourishing Nutty Delight	Chia Berry Smoothie Bowl	Green Detox Smoothie	Vegan Chickpea Omelette	Sunny Quinoa Bowl
Lunch	Spicy Avocado and Chickpea Sandwich	Grilled Shrimp with Rosemary Lemon Sauce	Quinoa Stuffed Bell Peppers	Tuna Nicoise Salad	Pan-Seared Cod with Sautéed Spinach	Eggplant and Chickpea Stew	Veggie Hummus Wrap
Snack	Creamy Avocado Dip	Baked Zucchini Chips	Refreshing Watermelon Salad	Roasted Red Pepper Hummus	Toasted Pumpkin Seeds	Grilled Pineapple Spears	Tangy Greek Yogurt Dip
Dinner	Chicken Marsala with Sautéed Mushrooms	Grilled Tuna Steaks with Citrus Glaze	Veggie Tofu Stir-fry	Grilled Lemon-Thyme Lamb Chops	Lemon and Dill Baked Cod	Quinoa and Lentil Salad	Italian-Style Beef Ragu

Chapter 13: Feasting without Fear: Holiday and Special Occasion Guide

---

13.1. Navigating Parties and Buffets

We've come a long way on our journey toward understanding the nuances of the renal diet. Now, it's time to tackle one of the most challenging aspects of any diet—social events. Parties and buffets are commonplace in our social life and present a unique challenge for individuals following a strict dietary regimen.

The Deceptive Layout: Understanding the Buffet Spread

The allure of a buffet is unquestionable. With its vast array of dishes, catering to a symphony of tastes, it's a food lover's paradise. However, for those corralling their dietary needs, a buffet can cloak potential dietary hazards under the guise of variety and freedom.

Understanding the layout of the buffet spread can be an invaluable strategy to maintain control amid the smorgasbord of dishes. First, conduct a thorough visual survey of the food array before picking up a plate. Identifying what foods align with your diet and which to avoid means half your battle is already won.

The Power of Selection: Making the Right Choice

The cornerstone of successfully navigating a buffet lies in exercising the power of selection – choosing the right foods that coincide with your dietary restrictions. A typical buffet range has a balance of vegetables, lean meats, seafood, and carbohydrates. As a person adhering to a renal diet, you should ideally opt for fresh vegetables, lean proteins, and whole-grain food options.

Avoiding dishes that are cream-based, fried, or dressed extravagantly is a prudent choice - these fancy deceptions often carry hidden sodium, potassium, and phosphorus.

Moderation: Taming the Portion Monster

Buffets are synonymous with abundance, which often leads us into another potential trap — overeating. Using smaller plates can trick your mind into thinking you're consuming a lot when you're not. Moreover, don't forget to assign half your plate to vegetables, followed by a quarter each for proteins and carbohydrates.

Remember, subscribing to a renal diet does not mean you can't relish the buffet norms. You can still explore variety and depth in flavors — the key is to make mindful choices and have control over your portions.

Appetizers and Desserts: Treading the Culinary Extremes

At the extremes of the buffet table, lie the appetizers and desserts, both posing unique dietary challenges. Appetizers often precede the main course, and since one usually approaches them with an appetite, these can be a slippery slope. Opt for something light and fresh, perhaps a salad or grapes, to check that hunger without a profound impact on your dietary balance. Beware of sodium-packed bites or creamy sauces.

As for desserts, a common pitfall at the end of the buffet line, you can seek fruit-based options or, even better, a fresh fruit salad. However, always be cautious of any added sugars or creams. Keep portions small and ensure you do not stray far from your renal diet parameters, even when faced with the sweetest temptation.

A Strategy for All Parties: Bringing Your Own Dish

A strategy that has proved beneficial for many on specialized diets is bringing their own dish to parties. This serves a dual purpose. Firstly, you can guarantee there's at least one dish you can freely enjoy without compromising your renal diet. Secondly, it can spark conversations about your dietary journey, enlightening others about the renal diet. Who knows? Your contribution might turn out to be the hit of the party!

13.2. Adapting Traditional Meals to the Renal Diet

The joyous times of the year, filled with tradition, memories, and familiar flavors, are often centered around food. These special meals are more than just nourishment—they are ties to our past, celebrations of the present, and even aspirations for the future. It's a time when the aroma of an age-old family recipe can flow through the house, summoning feelings of warmth, love, memory, and anticipation. However, when you're on a renal diet, these traditions can seem daunting.

"Fear not," we say, for adapting traditional meals to your renal diet is more within your reach than you might imagine. You can still partake in the joy of holiday feasting—just with a twist.

A New Lens on Familiar Flavors

Your time-honored family recipes might appear off-limits because they contain ingredients high in sodium, potassium, or phosphorus. However, it's important to remember that just as each family has its unique traditions, each recipe has unique adaptable potential too.

Let's consider the classic holiday roast, notoriously high in sodium and often prepared with high-phosphorus gravy. By eschewing the premade mixes and whipping up your homemade gravy using low-sodium broth, you can serve a delicious roast aligned with your renal parameters. Additions of herbs and spices like rosemary, garlic, and black pepper can compensate for the lack of salt, bringing in a depth of flavor that your taste buds will cherish.

The Substitution Game

While revitalizing family recipes for a renal diet, the art of substitution becomes your best friend. With careful swaps, you can not only tick to the tune of your dietary restrictions but also discover new gustatory territories.

Take the classic mashed potato, usually laden with heavy cream and an abundance of salt. By using garlic, olive oil, and a touch of the right kind of cheese, you can still prepare a creamy, flavorful side without the excessive potassium and sodium.

When it comes to desserts, reducing sugars and using kidney-friendly alternatives as sweeteners can produce light, delicious results. For instance, that beloved pumpkin pie? Baking a renal-friendly version means reducing the sugar, using an egg substitute, and creating a crust out of low-phosphorus materials. Your taste buds would barely notice the changes, but your kidneys certainly will.

Imagine, being able to savor your family fare, now transformed into your very own collection of kidney-friendly recipes.

Navigating Seafood Traditions

Seafood has been a center of festive dining across cultures and generations. Yet those on a renal diet often remain skeptical, given seafood's reputation for high phosphorus levels. But let's step back a little. Not all seafood is created equal when it comes to phosphorus content. For instance, crab, lobster, and shrimp are much lower in phosphorus as compared to other seafood, making them a possible part of your holiday menu.

A culinary tip here: While preparing your seafood dish, cook with fresh lemon juice, an array of herbs, or a butter substitute with less sodium. Not only would this match your renal diet, but would also lend a gourmet touch to your festivities.

Adapting meals to your renal diet is not a journey you take away from your heritage but towards it. It's about reshaping our notion of tradition, from being something we simply inherit and reenact to something we consciously mold and redefine for our well-being. It is about preserving the essence of the tradition, and yet striving for a future where we keep securing our health and happiness.

So, remember, each traditional meal you adapt to your renal diet is not just a victory for responsible eating, but also a fresh chapter in your family history, waiting to be passed down to the generations to come.

13.3. Dining Out on a Renal Diet

Eating at restaurants and attending social gatherings involving meals can be a challenge for the renal community. By following a few simple steps and empowering yourself with knowledge, dining out can become a pleasurable and satisfying experience once again.

Becoming a Savvy Diner

Prior to stepping out for a meal, some research will go a long way to ensure a delightful outcome. Look for restaurants that offer a diverse selection of renal-friendly ingredients and are willing to accommodate special requests. Checking menus online and calling the restaurant in advance can help you identify the establishments best suited to meet your needs.

Once you've chosen your dining destination, be mindful of the timing—you don't want to arrive during peak hours when the kitchen is swamped, and chefs may not have the flexibility to cater to special requests. Aim for earlier or later dining times when the staff will be more relaxed and able to accommodate your needs.

Getting to Know the Menu

Upon arrival, perusing the menu should be more than just a quick glance. Start by looking for dishes made with lean proteins and vegetables, while avoiding high-sodium, high-potassium, and high-phosphorus items.

Next, zero in on suitable dishes that require minimal modification, and keep an eye out for descriptors like "steamed," "grilled," or "broiled," which usually indicate healthier cooking methods. Avoid dishes featuring cream sauces, gravies, or excessive cheese, as these may contain hidden sources of sodium, potassium, or phosphorus.

It's okay to ask your server questions about the ingredients and preparation techniques used for your chosen dishes—after all, you're the customer, and the staff is there to help you have an enjoyable dining experience.

Customizing Your Order

When placing your order, gently inform your server about your dietary restrictions and ask for customized adjustments. While making your requests, be proactive by suggesting renal diet-friendly substitutions. For instance, in lieu of a high-sodium sauce, ask for a side of salsa, a fresh herb garnish, or a drizzle of heart-healthy olive oil.

If a dish calls for high-potassium ingredients such as tomatoes or potatoes, see if the kitchen can swap them out for lower-potassium alternatives. Perhaps even offering both options, like a veggie ratatouille made with bell peppers and zucchini or a cauliflower mashed potato, would delight your taste buds.

Additionally, it's always wise to confirm the portion sizes of your order. Ask the kitchen to serve a smaller, renal-diet appropriate portion if necessary, or consider sharing your dish with a dining partner.

Savoring Your Success

Navigating the world of dining out and buffets on a renal diet can be a gratifying adventure, particularly once you gain confidence in your ability to choose wisely and customize orders. Embrace these newfound skills with pride, as awareness and adaptability are the cornerstones to a successful renal journey.

As you continue to dine out and attend social events, you may wish to develop a list of your favorite restaurants and menu items that align with your renal diet requirements. In doing so, you'll be better-equipped to make informed, satisfying choices when dining out, and create a seamless experience that is as pleasurable as it is healthful.

So, instead of shying away from the opportunity to dine out or join friends and family at social events, face these experiences head-on, armed with the knowledge and strategies

gleaned from your journey through the renal diet. Remember, the more confident you are in your choices, the more enjoyable your experience will be—for you and those around you.

Chapter 14: Doctor Says: Frequently Asked Questions and Answers

1. Question: I've heard that all patients with kidney disease need to follow a low-protein diet. Is that accurate?

Answer: Not necessarily. The need for a low-protein diet depends on your kidney function, the cause of your kidney disease, and the recommendations of your healthcare provider. Each person is unique and nutritional needs can vary.

2. Question: Can excessive fluid intake worsen kidney function?

Answer: While hydration is important, for those with advanced kidney disease, fluid restriction might be necessary to prevent fluid buildup. Always consult with your healthcare provider to determine the right fluid intake for you.

3: Question: Are all fruits and vegetables beneficial for kidney health?

Answer: While fruits and vegetables offer plentiful health benefits, those with kidney disease may need to avoid those high in potassium such as bananas, oranges, potatoes, and tomatoes.

4. Question: Is it true that dairy products are bad for kidney health?

Answer: Dairy products can contribute to the intake of phosphorus, a mineral that kidneys struggle to process in the later stages of kidney diseases. However, not all dairy products have the same impact, so moderation and careful selection are key.

5. Question: Can processed foods be part of a kidney-friendly diet?

Answer: Processed foods tend to be high in sodium and phosphorus additives, both of which can be challenging for compromised kidneys. It's generally recommended to limit consumption of these products.

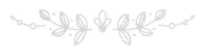

6. Question: I enjoy a glass of wine occasionally—is alcohol entirely off-limits?

Answer: Occasional moderate intake may be permissible, but it's crucial to consult your healthcare provider as alcohol can affect blood pressure, liver, and fluid balance.

7. Question: Do renal patients always require potassium and phosphorus restrictions?

Answer: Not all patients require these restrictions. It's usually needed for those with advanced kidney disease or those on dialysis. Regular blood tests guide these dietary adjustments.

8. Question: I have diabetes and kidney disease – can I still have fruits?

Answer: Yes, but the choice of fruits must take into consideration both kidney and blood sugar control, necessitating a careful selection of low-potassium, low-sugar fruits.

9. Question: Are plant-based proteins better than animal proteins for kidney health?

Answer: Plant-based proteins can be easier on the kidneys and beneficial for overall health. However, they must be used cautiously in renal diets due to their potassium content.

10. Question: Can food seasoning affect my renal diet?

Answer: Yes, many seasonings contain sodium. Opt for fresh herbs, spices, and salt substitutes that don't compromise your kidney health.

11. Question: Is a renal diet only beneficial for kidney disease patients?

Answer: A renal diet is structured primarily for those with kidney disease, but its principles of low-sodium, low processed foods, and balanced nutrient intake certainly benefit overall health.

12. Question: Can high blood pressure lead to kidney diseases?

Answer: Yes, hypertension can damage the kidneys over time, leading to kidney disease.

13. Question: Is caffeine harmful to my kidneys?

Answer: In moderation, caffeine poses no threat to kidney health. However, excessive consumption can raise blood pressure. Limit to 1-2 cups per day.

14. Question: Will the renal diet cure my kidney disease?

Answer: While a renal diet cannot reverse kidney disease, it can certainly slow disease progression, help manage symptoms, and improve overall health.

15. Question: I have kidney disease. Do I need to limit my physical activities?

Answer: On the contrary, physical activity is encouraged as it aids blood pressure control and overall wellness. Always consult with your healthcare provider about the types and amount of exercise suitable for you.

16. Question: How important is regular check-ups in managing kidney health?

Answer: Regular check-ups are crucial for managing kidney health. Kidney disease often progresses silently, and routine check-ups allow for early detection, which can help slow disease progression and manage symptoms more effectively. Your healthcare provider can monitor your blood pressure, test your blood for kidney function markers, and check your urine for protein, all of which are important indicators of kidney health. Regular appointments also give you an opportunity to discuss your diet and lifestyle choices and make any necessary adjustments. Remember, the earlier a problem is detected, the better it can be managed.

17. Question: I am overweight. Will losing weight improve my kidney health?

Answer: Weight loss can help control blood pressure and manage diabetes, both of which contribute to kidney disease.

18. Question: How critical is timing and frequency of meals, in kidney health?

Answer: Meal timing isn't as important as meal content. However, regular meals with controlled portions can prevent overeating and assist in managing blood sugar levels.

19. Question: Are high-fiber food beneficial for a renal diet?

Answer: Yes, but intake of high-fiber foods (like some fruits, vegetables, and whole grains) needs to be balanced with their potassium and phosphorus content.

20. Question: Are there any safe and beneficial supplements for someone with kidney disease?

Answer: Absolutely, there are some supplements that could potentially support kidney health, but it's important to choose them wisely and always under the supervision of healthcare professional.

-> **Omega-3 fatty acids:** Omega-3s are known for their anti-inflammatory properties which might help protect against progression of kidney disease. They also support heart health, which is important as heart disease is often linked with kidney disease.
Suggested Product: Nordic Naturals Omega-3 (https://amzn.to/40TfmKN)

->**Probiotics:** These can offer kidney health benefits by helping to control urea levels, a common complication for individuals with kidney issues. Probiotics also support overall digestive health.
Suggested Product: Renadyl Probiotics for Kidney Health (https://amzn.to/3GfMVob)

->**Chitosan:** Chitosan, a sugar extracted from the outer layers of seafood like lobsters, crabs, and shrimp, may help support kidney function by binding phosphorus in food.
Suggested Product: NOW Foods Chitosan (https://amzn.to/3QZsqd6)

Chapter 15: Keeping the Faith: Inspirational Stories of Success

15.1. Personal Stories of Overcoming Obstacles

The journey towards a healthy kidney lifestyle is often filled with challenges, but the strength and determination of individuals who have walked this path serve as an inspiration. It's important to remember that you are not alone in this journey, and the perseverance of others can provide motivation and encouragement. Let's explore some personal stories of overcoming obstacles and maintaining hope despite the challenges faced by those with kidney disease.

Maria's Triumph Over Adversity

Maria was a vibrant, energetic woman in her early 40s when she suddenly found out that she suffered from advanced kidney disease. Devastated by the news, she felt like her entire world had crumbled. But Maria refused to let her diagnosis define or limit her. Maria took the challenge head-on and embraced the renal diet, became more dedicated to her daily exercise, and began attending a support group for people with kidney disease.

Over time, Maria noticed a vast improvement in her kidney function and gained a sense of control over her health. Her story is one of resilience, serving as an inspiration to those also facing challenges. Through her unwavering determination, Maria proved that maintaining hope and adopting a positive attitude can make a significant difference when tackling obstacles in life.

Samuel's Journey to Self-Care

Samuel had always been the kind of person who prioritized everyone else's well-being over his own until his kidney disease diagnosis forced him to reevaluate his choices. With support from his family and friends, Samuel embraced self-care by prioritizing the renal diet and incorporating exercise into his daily routine. He no longer viewed caring for himself as selfish but understood it as a necessary aspect of maintaining his well-being.

By learning to listen to his body and make healthier choices, Samuel discovered the importance of self-care in recovering kidney health.

Sarah's Support Network

Sarah was 28 when she was diagnosed with kidney disease. Like many people confronted with a life-changing medical diagnosis, Sarah was initially overwhelmed by the unknown. In her case, she found solace in creating a strong support network of friends, family, and fellow kidney patients.

Sarah's support network played a crucial role in helping her navigate the complex world of kidney disease and the renal diet. Battling kidney disease alone can be an isolating experience, but Sarah's story demonstrates that surrounding yourself with people who understand your challenges can be an essential part of the journey.

Overcoming Obstacles Together

Each person's experience with kidney disease is unique, but these stories showcase the power of determination, resilience, and positivity in overcoming obstacles. Embracing a healthy renal diet, practicing self-care, and building a support network can provide strength and hope when facing challenges in life. By learning from these experiences and maintaining faith in ourselves and our abilities, we can continue to achieve success despite the adversities we face.

15.2. Tips for Staying Motivated

Set Realistic Goals and Celebrate Small Victories

It's essential to set achievable, realistic goals for yourself. Break down your long-term objectives into smaller, more manageable steps. This will give you a sense of progress and accomplishment, helping to maintain your motivation. Remember, small victories add up, and over time, they will make a significant impact on your health and well-being.

- **Find What Inspires You**

Inspiration can come in different forms, from motivational quotes and personal stories to pictures and mementos that remind you why you're on this journey. Surround yourself with things that inspire and motivate you to stay committed to your kidney health journey. Turn to these images or words when you need a boost of encouragement.

- **Keep a Journal**

Writing down your thoughts and emotions can provide significant benefits, especially during challenging times. Use your journal to document both short-term and long-term goals, as well as noting any achievements or improvements you've made along the way. By reflecting on your progress, you'll be more aware of your strengths and equipped to overcome future setbacks.

- **Make It Enjoyable**

Adopting a renal diet can feel restrictive, but it doesn't mean you have to sacrifice delicious meals or feel deprived. Find joy in discovering new, kidney-friendly recipes and experimenting with various herbs and spices to enhance the flavor of your dishes. By making your diet enjoyable, you'll be more likely to stick with it and remain motivated.

- **Embrace Self-Care**

Incorporating self-care into your routine is an essential part of staying motivated. Listening to your body's needs and prioritizing your physical and emotional well-being will help you maintain balance and encourage ongoing success. Make time for relaxation and stress-relief activities, such as walking, meditation, or hobbies that bring you joy.

In conclusion, staying motivated on your kidney health journey is crucial to achieving long-term success and a better quality of life.

Conclusion:

As we draw the curtain on our collective exploration of kidney health and the renal diet, I trust that you, dear reader, are stepping away equipped with knowledge, inspiration, and a heightened sense of empowerment. This journey has been one of understanding, adapting, and reclaiming control of your well-being.

This book was born out of my medical expertise, experiences, and my commitment to guiding individuals like you on the journey to improve kidney health. However, the completion of this book is not the termination of your journey; instead, it's the commencement of your personal exploration into the applications of this knowledge.

We have delved into the significance of kidney health, mastered permitted and prohibited foods, understood the art of cooking and seasoning, and savored a gamut of kidney-friendly, delightful recipes. We've shone a light on the fears of social dining, equipped you with the tools to navigate special occasions, and wrapped it all up with an inspiring demonstration of faith through stories of successful kidney health journeys.

As a nephrologist and guide in your journey, my hope is that this book serves as a steppingstone toward a kidney-friendly lifestyle, filling you with determination, courage, and optimism needed for the road ahead. I believe in you and your capability to successfully navigate this journey because you are now an informed advocate for your health.

Remember, your journey with the renal diet is not a punishment or a limitation, but rather an opportunity for creating a healthier, fulfilling life in harmony with your unique dietary requirements. With this spirit, I bid you a confident, fervent journey ahead, trusting that this book will remain a constant, reliable companion in your quest for better kidney health.

Dr. Tamara S. Kears